Living with Opioids

Julie R. Gaither

Living with Opioids

A Clarion Call to Safeguarding our Homes and Families

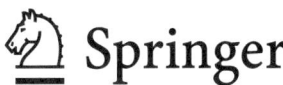

Julie R. Gaither
Department of Pediatrics
Yale School of Medicine
New Haven, CT, USA

ISBN 978-3-031-95819-9   ISBN 978-3-031-95820-5 (eBook)
https://doi.org/10.1007/978-3-031-95820-5

© The Editor(s) (if applicable) and The Author(s), under exclusive license to Springer Nature Switzerland AG 2026

This work is subject to copyright. All rights are solely and exclusively licensed by the Publisher, whether the whole or part of the material is concerned, specifically the rights of translation, reprinting, reuse of illustrations, recitation, broadcasting, reproduction on microfilms or in any other physical way, and transmission or information storage and retrieval, electronic adaptation, computer software, or by similar or dissimilar methodology now known or hereafter developed.
The use of general descriptive names, registered names, trademarks, service marks, etc. in this publication does not imply, even in the absence of a specific statement, that such names are exempt from the relevant protective laws and regulations and therefore free for general use.
The publisher, the authors and the editors are safe to assume that the advice and information in this book are believed to be true and accurate at the date of publication. Neither the publisher nor the authors or the editors give a warranty, expressed or implied, with respect to the material contained herein or for any errors or omissions that may have been made. The publisher remains neutral with regard to jurisdictional claims in published maps and institutional affiliations.

This Springer imprint is published by the registered company Springer Nature Switzerland AG
The registered company address is: Gewerbestrasse 11, 6330 Cham, Switzerland

If disposing of this product, please recycle the paper.

Dedicated to my parents, J.D. "Jake" and Rozelle Gaither

Preface

In 2019, I wrote an op-ed for the *Hartford Courant* urging families to start taking a more active role in protecting themselves from opioids. I outlined what I saw as a fundamental failure on the part of the government, public health officials, and researchers to educate families about the dangers of opioids and the practical measures they could take to protect themselves.

At the time, I had been researching the opioid epidemic for nearly a decade and was struck by how little children factored into the national conversation surrounding opioids. At least 10,000 children had died from opioid poisonings in the span of just 20 years. I acknowledged that it would be easy to dismiss these deaths given the hundreds of thousands of adults who had lost their lives during this time, but I also asked the public to consider whether focusing on children might in fact be the key to containing the worst drug crisis in this country's history. I asked the public to consider whether commonsense measures that we think of as applicable mainly to children could also save adult lives.

In the seven years since this piece was published, this question has only increased in urgency. Despite hundreds of policies, procedures, laws, and regulations aimed at containing the crisis, the death toll continues to mount. To date, more than 600,000 adults have died from fatal opioid overdoses and another 5000 children have died from poisonings—bringing the total to at least 15,000 children.

And yet, so little has changed in our response to the crisis, which continues to focus primarily on adults in isolation of their families and ignoring a central truth: the home is where the struggle with opioid use, addiction, and recovery takes place. Contrary to public perception, most people who die from opioids don't die "on the street," they die at home. This is true for both children and for adults.

Physicians are prescribing opioids less frequently, but only moderately so. The most recent estimate is that nationwide doctors write about 38 prescriptions for every 100 people in the United States, and in certain areas of the country, this number is far higher. In Alabama and Arkansas, for example, 72 prescriptions are written for every 100 residents.

Perhaps more important, there has been no substantial change to opioid packaging in the way of making them safer for children. While the Poisoning Prevention Packaging Act requires child-resistant packaging for most oral prescription medications, manufacturers are able to provide non-child-resistant ("adult friendly") packaging if requested by the prescribing doctor or the patient. This is true even for opioid medications known to be life-threatening to young children because of their potency, pharmacological makeup, or long-acting nature. Suboxone, for example, is a long-acting opioid primarily used to treat opioid use disorder. Yet, it comes packaged in a foil wrapper, and the medication itself is brightly colored and could be mistaken for candy by a child. Likewise, Duragesic transdermal patches deliver round-the-clock fentanyl to patients with chronic pain over the course of several days, but there have been numerous cases of children dying after coming into contact with discarded patches. There have even been cases of children dying after being exposed to a patch being worn by an adult.

Remarkably, there has been little change in the labeling of prescription opioids. Currently, only three states—Arizona, Hawaii, and Connecticut—require pharmacists to affix warning labels to opioids, and in New Jersey and New York, legislation has recently been introduced that would make warning labels a requirement. In general, these labels address the risks of overdose and addiction. Only in Connecticut, my home state, do the labels warn of the risks that opioids pose to children: as of January 1, 2024, all opioids must come with a fluorescent orange sticker that reads, "DANGER TO CHILDREN. KEEP OUT OF REACH." To date, there is no evidence that similar labels will be required nationally by the Food and Drug Administration.

Few families receive instruction on proper storage or disposal of these medications. Fewer still understand what to do if a child is poisoned or an adult overdoses.

But, as most of us now know, prescription opioids are no longer the primary driver of the opioid crisis. Fentanyl, a synthetic opioid that is increasingly produced illegally, now accounts for more than 70% of all opioid deaths in adults and, astonishingly, 95% of all opioid deaths in children. In all, more than 5000 children have died from fentanyl over the past 25 years. The majority of these deaths, however, have occurred since 2013. Since that time, there has been a 3000% increase in pediatric deaths from fentanyl. Yet even though fentanyl has been a serious threat to the young in this country for nearly a decade, it was not until 2023 with the death of Nicholas Dominici, a 22-month-old who died from fentanyl exposure at a Bronx daycare where illegal drugs were being stored and sold, that the risk of fentanyl to children received national attention.

I had hoped that the death of this young child would be a turning point in the fight to bring awareness to how the young in this country have been overlooked regarding opioids. Instead, it was just one more story of someone dying from these toxic drugs. As one long-term resident of the community told BBC news, "It's sad that a little boy lost his life, but that's just an everyday thing."

Within the medical community, there has certainly been a shift in recent years, but this is primarily among researchers, clinicians, and child welfare workers who care for adolescents and families affected by substance use. Among the larger medical community, including among those who prescribe opioids for the treatment of opioid use disorder in adults, there is less awareness. And I argue that the broader lay public continues to be largely unaware of the dangers that opioids pose to themselves and their families even though opioids are embedded in American society and will remain so for the foreseeable future.

Thirty years after the crisis began, no one—parent or not—should lack a basic understanding of opioids risks, how they should be stored, and what to do with them when they are no longer needed. Every household should have a plan for responding if the worst happens—a child is poisoned or an adult overdoses.

My goal with this book, written for healthcare professionals, government officials, and the general public, is to shift the current paradigm from one that focuses only on adults to a more systemic, family-centered perspective. It is in the home where opioid exposures happen, where prevention is possible, and where common-sense solutions are likely to have an immediate impact.

In the pages that follow, I provide both an overview of what I have learned about opioids from my research—specifically, how they have harmed us—and, more important, what we must do to keep ourselves safe. I present a brief historical account of opioids in American society, focusing on past efforts to limit their harms. I also share the most current research on the state of the crisis, where we've made advances (such as with the availability of over-the-counter naloxone), and where we have fallen short. I present practical steps that families with the support of their healthcare providers can take to protect themselves. I explore what we can learn from peer nations in how they have managed to avoid the devastation seen in this country. Finally, I look to the future and how we can use the opioid settlement funds to begin prioritizing children and families in our efforts to mitigate the harms caused by these drugs.

This book is about more than opioids. It is about our capacity to care for vulnerable families, particularly those affected by substance use, and how to help them care for themselves. By returning to foundational principles of child safety and family well-being, we can not only address today's opioid crisis but also build stronger defenses against the future threats that opioids and other substances will surely bring.

New Haven, CT, USA   Julie R. Gaither

Acknowledgments

Thank you to Gregory Sutorius, my editor at Springer, for his patience as I worked through writing this—my first book. Thank you to Steve Aitken, who copyedited the manuscript and provided reassurance when I needed it most.

Thank you to my colleagues at Yale: Linda Mayes, Kirsten Bechtel, Veronika Shabanova, Matthew Grossman, Gunjan Tiyyagura, Deepa Camenga, and my research assistants, Dara Gleeson and Yi Li. A special thank you to John Leventhal, my mentor for the past 15 years.

Thank you to Debra Gregory and Jenny Peek for their support over the years.

Thank you to my mother, Rozelle Gaither, and my late father, J. D. Gaither, who asked me repeatedly: "Julie, do you know how to write a book?" For him, I learned how.

Thank you to my family for their unwavering support and reading nearly everything I have written over the years, no matter how technical: Becky Gaither, Eva Gaither Eff, Julianna Ruben, Rick Eff, Rakesh Sonker, and Lucas, Ryan, and Sydney DeCastilhos.

Lastly, thank you to Flavio DeCastilhos, my partner, for reading the book so closely and asking the best questions.

Contents

1	**Opioids Through History: The Unfulfilled Promise**	1
	1.1 From Opium to Morphine: The Initial Search for a Safe Opioid	1
	1.2 Heroin: The First "Nonaddictive" Alternative	2
	1.3 Early Regulation	3
	1.4 The Porter and Jick Letter: How Five Sentences Changed American Medicine	3
	1.5 "Pain as the 5th Vital Sign"	6
	1.6 OxyContin: A New Drug, a Deadly Crisis	7
	References	10
2	**The US Opioid Epidemic: An Evolving and Systemic Crisis**	11
	2.1 The Aftermath of OxyContin: From Regional Hot Spots to National Crisis	11
	2.2 Rising Availability and Deaths: The First Wave	13
	2.3 Unintended Consequences: The Reformulation of OxyContin	14
	2.4 The Second Wave: Heroin Fills the Prescription Void	15
	2.5 Fentanyl: The Third and Deadliest Wave	16
	2.6 Changing Demographics: From White Men to Minorities, Women, and Children	17
	2.7 Social Determinants and Vulnerable Populations	18
	References	19
3	**Neonatal Opioid Withdrawal Syndrome: Clinical Challenges and Evolving Approaches to Care**	21
	3.1 Understanding Neonatal Opioid Withdrawal Syndrome	21
	3.2 The Clinical and Economic Impact of NOWS	22
	3.3 Beyond the Hospital: Long-Term Challenges for Infants with NOWS	23
	3.4 Evolving Standards of Care: From Finnegan to Family-Centered Approaches	25
	3.5 The Eat, Sleep, Console Approach: A Paradigm Shift	26
	3.6 Research Gaps and Future Directions	28

	3.7	Toward Integrated Care Models: Supporting the Mother-Infant Dyad	30
	References		33
4	**The Hidden Crisis: How the Opioid Epidemic Has Endangered America's Children**		**35**
	4.1	The Overlooked Victims	35
	4.2	Changing Patterns in Pediatric Opioid Exposures	38
	4.3	Understanding How Children Die: Circumstances and Classifications	45
	4.4	Case Study: Marcello's Preventable Death	46
	4.5	System Failures and Missed Opportunities	48
	4.6	Implications for Policy and Practice	50
	References		51
5	**A Systemic Crisis: Failed Responses and Overlooked Solutions**		**53**
	5.1	The Fragmented Response: Individual Solutions for a Family Problem	53
	5.2	Failed Policy Initiatives	54
	5.3	Poor Quality of Care: Failure to Follow Prescribing Guidelines	55
	5.4	The Heightened Risks of Opioids for Patients with Substance Use Disorders	56
	5.5	Racial Disparities in Opioid Monitoring	57
	5.6	Regulatory Failures	58
	5.7	The Unintended Consequence of Changes to Methadone Policy During COVID	58
	5.8	Practices That Prioritize Adults Over Children	59
	5.9	Child Protection Policies: The Inadequacy of Plans of Safe Care	60
	5.10	Healthcare Provider Knowledge Gaps and Displacement of Responsibility	60
	5.11	Emergency Preparedness and Public Health Messaging	61
	5.12	Multi-level Prevention Strategies	63
	5.13	Research and Surveillance: Gaps in Knowledge	64
	References		65
6	**Ground Zero: Learning to Live with Opioids in Our Homes and Communities**		**69**
	6.1	A Family-Focused Framework	69
	6.2	A Child-Centered Approach That Benefits Everyone	70
	6.3	Education: What Families Need to Know	70
	6.4	Enhancing Provider Education to Support Families	71
	6.5	Practical Home-Safety Measures	73
		6.5.1 Safe Storage: Barriers to Access	74
		6.5.2 Safe Disposal: Removing Unnecessary Risks from the Home	75

| | | 6.5.3 Emergency Preparedness: When Prevention Fails. . . . . | 76 |
| | References. . . . . | 77 |

7 Strengthening the Safety Net: Institutional Approaches to Family Protection 79
   7.1 Beyond Individual Households: Supporting and Reinforcing Family Efforts. 79
   7.2 A Simple Checklist for a Complex Problem 80
   7.3 Healthcare Systems Integration: Embedding Safety at Every Point of Contact 81
   7.4 Evidence-Based Quality of Care and Monitoring 82
   7.5 Community-Based Support Networks. 83
   7.6 Regulatory Approaches: Designing Safety into Products and Systems. 83
   7.7 Family-Centered Addiction Treatment and Integrated Models 85
   References. 87

8 What Can We Learn from Other Countries, Past Eras? 91
   8.1 Global Perspectives: Learning from International Approaches to Opioid Safety. 91
   8.2 The Widening Gap: How the Opioid Crisis Exacerbates America's Health Disparities. 92
   8.3 Controlled Prescribing Practices 92
   8.4 Structure of Healthcare Systems and Universal Insurance Coverage 94
   8.5 Addiction Treatment Integration and Provider Training 95
   8.6 Cultural Factors 96
   8.7 Historical Perspectives: America's Changing Approach 96
   8.8 Lessons from Other Countries and the Past. 97
   References. 98

9 Opioid Settlement Funds: An Opportunity for States to Prioritize Children. 101
   9.1 National Opioid Litigation and Settlements 101
   9.2 The Framework: Distribution of Funds and Mechanisms for Oversight 102
   9.3 Funding Priorities: Five Guiding Principles and Nine Core Strategies 103
   9.4 Vulnerable Populations 104
   9.5 Promising Approaches: The Wisconsin Case Study 104
   9.6 The Critical Gaps. 105
   References. 108

10 Conclusion 109

Index. 111

Abbreviations and Acronyms

AAP	American Academy of Pediatrics
ACT NOW	Advancing Clinical Trials for Neonatal Opioid Withdrawal
CDC	Centers for Disease Control and Prevention
CAPTA	Child Abuse Prevention and Treatment Act
CPS	Child Protective Services
CPR	Cardiopulmonary Resuscitation
CPSC	Consumer Product Safety Commission
DCF	Department of Children and Families
DEA	Drug Enforcement Administration
DSM-5	*Diagnostic Statistical Manual*, fifth edition
FBR	Family-Based Recovery
FDA	Food and Drug Administration
FNAST	Finnegan Neonatal Abstinence Scoring Tool
ESC	Eat, Sleep, Console
HHS	Department of Health and Human Services
IMF	Illegally Manufactured Fentanyl
JCAHO	Joint Commission on Accreditation of Hospital Organizations
KIDOs	Kids in Danger of Opioids
MAT	Medication-Assisted Treatment
MMEs	Milligrams of Morphine Equivalents
MMT	Methadone Maintenance Treatment
MOMs	Maternal Overdose Matters
MIO	Mothering from the Inside Out
NAS	Neonatal Abstinence Syndrome
NEJM	*New England Journal of Medicine*
NICU	Neonatal Intensive Care Unit
NIH	National Institutes of Health
NOWS	Neonatal Opioid Withdrawal Syndrome
NSDUH	National Survey on Drug Use and Health
OB-GYN	Obstetrics and Gynecology
OBOE	Outcomes of Babies with Opioid Exposure
OCA	Office of the Child Advocate
OUD	Opioid Use Disorder

POSC	Plans of Safe Care
PPPA	Poison Prevention Packaging Act
SAMHSA	Substance Abuse and Mental Health Services Administration
WHO	World Health Organization

Opioids Through History: The Unfulfilled Promise

The opioid epidemic stands alone as the defining public health crisis of our modern era, but America's struggle with opioids and the opium plant from which it is derived dates back centuries. To comprehend the current crisis and how opioids became the leading cause of injury in the United States—surpassing even deaths from motor vehicle accidents—it is necessary to understand opioids through a historical lens. Much of what we struggle with today is not new, and many of our efforts to control opioids' harms have historical precedents. This chapter traces opium's journey to North America in the 1600s, through the development of morphine and heroin (initially marketed as "a safe family drug") in the 1800s, to the introduction of OxyContin in 1996. Throughout these historical eras, a consistent pattern emerges: the pursuit of a nonaddictive opioid—what has been called the "holy grail of pain medicine"—has repeatedly ended in crisis.

1.1   From Opium to Morphine: The Initial Search for a Safe Opioid

It took thousands of years for opium to reach North America, where colonists in the 1600s mixed it with alcohol to create laudanum [1]. By the early nineteenth century, opium-laced syrups were used to induce euphoria, treat anxiety, and soothe pain, including menstrual cramps in women and teething pain in babies [2]. But opium was potent and unpredictable.

In a search to find an alternative to opium that would produce the same benefits but in a more controlled form, a young pharmacist's apprentice in Germany, Friedrich Wilhelm Adam Sertürner, isolated the drug's active compound in 1803 [3]. He called it "morphine," after the Greek god of dreams [2]. Morphine was heralded as reliable, long-lasting, and, above all, safe. But soon, "God's own medicine," as it was called by physicians, was found to be highly addictive [4].

1.2 Heroin: The First "Nonaddictive" Alternative

It is here in history that the quest by the pharmaceutical industry to find what Travis Rieder of the Berman Institute of Bioethics has called "the holy grail of pain medicine"—a nonaddictive opioid—began in earnest [2]. Heroin, which was discovered in the 1870s, was initially thought to be such a drug. It was discovered by an English chemist, C.R. Alder Wright, who created the drug by boiling morphine with acetic anhydride (a compound that 20 years later would be used to synthesize aspirin).

In 1898, the Bayer company introduced the derivative of morphine discovered by Wright and called it "heroin" after the German word *heroisch*, which translates to "heroic" in English. Heroin was marketed as a pain remedy and cough suppressant that was safe even for infants. Bayer associates called it "A safe family drug" that was "doctor-approved" [5]. It was often used to treat the symptoms of disease common at the time, including tuberculosis. Heroin was stronger than morphine, also cheaper, and for a time it was thought to be less addictive. But this was soon proven wrong. Doctors discovered that patients quickly grew dependent upon the elixir and increasingly needed stronger and stronger doses, and soon heroin was being used recreationally in large cities.

Doctors and laypersons alike were free to use the drugs to treat everyday conditions as they saw fit. But in the late 1800s, there was a shift underfoot, which is reflected in the 1888 publication by James Adams, a physician in Massachusetts, in *The Boston Medical and Surgical Journal*, which would later become *The New England Journal of Medicine (NEJM)* [6]. Referring to opium specifically, Adams wrote:

> Opium is the most conspicuous article in the pharmacopeia. Its extraordinary efficacy in relieving pain, the versatility of its powers, and its reliability in emergencies, give it preeminent standing. It is generally recognized by the medical profession as the most indispensable of drugs. But, while surpassing other remedies in its beneficent effects, it is remarkable in its power for harm. Hence, its medical use requires a degree of caution not less than that with which the surgeon handles the scalpel. When to administer and when to withhold it, constitute one of the gravest of medical problems. There are times when the dangers and disadvantages of this most brilliant of drugs seem wholly out of proportion to its benefits. A growing dissatisfaction with opium is the motive of the present paper, which is designed as an argument in favor of restricting the use of opiates to a greater degree than has hitherto been the prevailing custom. The disadvantages of opium are these: (1) In an overdose it is an active poison. (2) In ordinary doses its benefits are largely offset by various functional derangements. (3) Its use involves the danger of the opium-habit.

And in a passage that could have been written about the modern-day opioid epidemic, Adams writes:

> It has been charged that the medical profession is largely responsible for the prevalence of the opium-habit. That some cases do result from opiate prescriptions cannot be denied; but it is my belief that, in the practice of educated and respectable medical men, such occurrences are very rare. Physicians are incessantly warning their patients against the dangers of, and, as a rule, administer this drug with the utmost caution. The prime causes of the opium-habit are undoubtedly to be found in the unrestricted sale of opiates….The avidity

with which the new analgesics are seized upon by the medical profession and their powers tested is an indication of the deep-seated antipathy to opium, and the desire to be emancipated from its rule.

1.3 Early Regulation

Up until the early 1900s, there was limited oversight in how drugs such as morphine and heroin were used, but in 1906 the Pure Food and Drug Act required that the active ingredients be listed in medications [2]. The 1914 Harrison Narcotic Act soon followed, which "taxed and regulated the industry," requiring anyone dealing in opiates to be registered. The goal, according to Dr. David Courtwright, a historian on US drug history, was to control and limit the distribution of opiates. A decade later, heroin was made illegal in the United States with the passage of the Heroin Act of 1924, which prohibited the production, possession, or use—even for medical purposes—of heroin (Bayer had ceased producing the drug in 1913). To further control opioid prescribing in the United States, in 1930 the Federal Bureau of Narcotics was founded. All told, these federal regulations served to tamp down the use and abuse of prescription opioids but provided fuel for illicit use. Heroin use exploded in large urban areas, such as New York City, in the 1960s. Echoing the current epidemic, heroin use was largely fueled by addiction among young men.

The next decade brought about the Controlled Substances Act of 1970, which classified psychoactive drugs into five categories based on effectiveness and risks, including addiction risk. By the time that Percocet and Vicodin came on the market in the late 1970s, it was ingrained in doctors that prescribing opioids should be avoided because they were so highly addictive.

1.4 The Porter and Jick Letter: How Five Sentences Changed American Medicine

But had the pendulum swung too far? Inevitably a few doctors in the 1970s and 1980s began pushing back, questioning the "conservative prescribing norms" [2]. Critics of the restrictions placed on opioids frequently cited a letter to the editor of the *NEJM* [2]. Published in January 10, 1980, the letter, written by Jane Porter and Dr. Hershel Jick, was titled "Addiction Rare in Patients Treated with Narcotics" [7]. The letter consisted of one paragraph—five sentences in all:

> To the Editor: Recently, we examined our current files to determine the incidence of narcotic addiction in 39,946 hospitalized medical patients who were monitored consecutively. Although there were 11,882 patients who received at least one narcotic preparation, there were only four cases of reasonably well documented addiction in patients who had no history of addiction. The addiction was considered major in only one instance. The drugs implicated were meperidine in two patients, Percodan in one, and hydromorphone in one. We conclude that despite widespread use of narcotics drugs in hospitals, the development of addiction is rare in medical patients with no history of addiction.

There was no evidence provided in support of the data and only two citations were given. And yet, the letter was widely invoked to support the claim that using opioids for the treatment of chronic pain carried little risk of addiction. What most supporters chose to ignore—intentionally or not—was that the patients noted in the letter were *hospitalized*, meaning these were patients who were observed in a controlled environment and followed for a short period of time. Chronic pain is just that—chronic—and its management with opioids requires their use over a long period of time, typically months if not years (long-term opioid therapy is standardly defined as more than 90 days of consecutive treatment).

Today, there is an editor's note attached to the Porter and Jick letter that states: "For reasons of public health, readers should be aware that this letter has been 'heavily and uncritically' cited as evidence that addiction is rare with opioid therapy. Leung et al. describe its history."

The Leung citation is in reference to another *NEJM* letter to the editor. Published in June 2017, it outlines a study conducted by a team of researchers in Canada [8]. Pamela T.M. Leung of the University of Toronto and colleagues analyzed 608 journal articles that followed the original 1980 letter and categorized each of the citations as either affirming or negating the claim made in the 1980 letter that "the development of addiction is rare in medical patients with no history of addiction." The vast majority of articles supported the conclusion made by Porter and Jick. In fact, 72% of articles cited the letter as evidence that opioid addiction was rare. Astoundingly, 80% failed to note that the patients described in the letter were hospitalized. Leung et al. go on to note that there was a "sizable increase" in publications citing the original 1980 letter around the time that OxyContin was introduced in 1996 (Fig. 1.1).

In their analysis of the articles that had cited the 1980 Porter and Jick paper, Leung et al. included select quotes from these articles to underscore the lack of equipoise (a state of professional uncertainty about the benefits and risks of treatment options) [9] that was displayed by the authors of these studies: "The pain population with no abuse history is literally at no risk for addiction," states a 1998 article published in the journal *Nursing Economics* titled "What is the Issue?: pseudoaddiction or the undertreatment of pain" [10]. And in an article published in the journal *The Independent Review* in 2006 (several years after the opioid crisis began), the author states, "In truth, however, the medical evidence overwhelmingly indicates that properly administered opioid therapy rarely if ever results in 'accidental addiction' or 'opioid abuse'" [11]. Leung et al. conclude their study by stating that the "citation pattern contributed to the North American opioid crisis by helping to shape a narrative that allayed prescribers' concerns about the risk of addiction associated with long-term opioid therapy."

Among those using the Porter and Jick paper to support the narrative that opioids were nonaddictive was the company Purdue Pharma, the makers of OxyContin, a high-dose and extended-release version of oxycodone, a drug that had been around since the early 1900s when it was discovered by two German chemists. Purdue, in developing OxyContin from oxycodone, a drug that in itself was twice as potent as morphine, was to completely upend the paradigm surrounding the treatment of pain

1.4 The Porter and Jick Letter: How Five Sentences Changed American Medicine

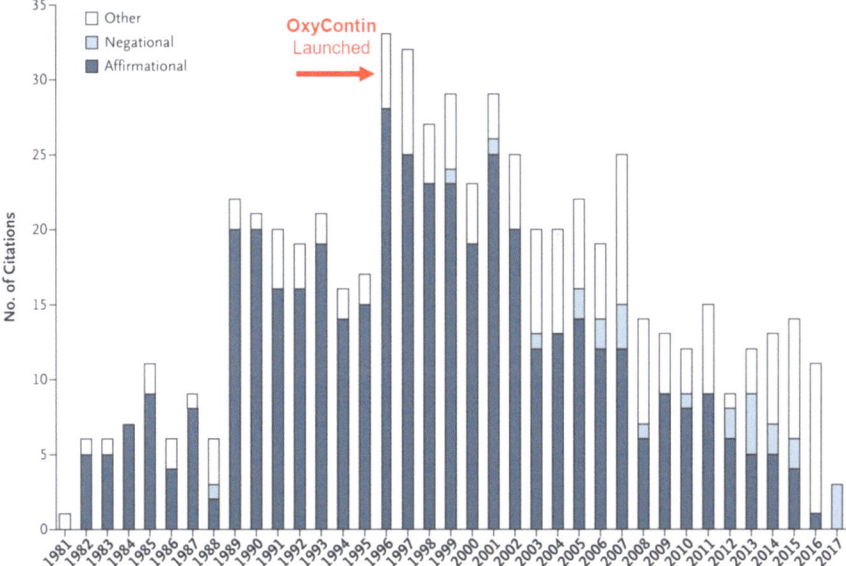

Fig. 1.1 Number and type of citations of the 1980 letter, according to year. Shown are number of citations of a 1980 letter to the *Journal* in which the correspondents claimed that opioid therapy rarely resulted in addiction. The citations are categorized according to whether the authors of the articles affirmed or negated the correspondents' conclusion about opioids. (Source: Leung et al. [8]. Copyright New England Journal of Medicine)

[12]. Prior to the 1990s, opioids were primarily restricted to treating end-of-life pain among patients with cancer, but OxyContin was conceived as a drug for anyone who suffered from chronic pain, not only those with cancer pain. Cancer pain was too niche a market; the real targets were those suffering from chronic, nonmalignant pain for conditions such as rheumatoid arthritis, osteoarthritis, fibromyalgia, back pain, and sickle cell anemia. According to Patrick Radden Keefe, the author of *Empire of Pain: The Secret History of the Sackler Dynasty*, the head of marketing at Purdue, Michael Friedman, envisioned marketing OxyContin to "*all* those patients" [12]. Friedman noted that four million prescriptions were written each year for cancer pain. At the time it was estimated that some 50 million Americans suffered from chronic noncancer pain, an enormous untapped market [12].

Purdue was helped along by several prominent organizations and individuals advocating for the use of opioids for both cancer and noncancer pain. The argument was that to withhold the drugs would be inhumane. In particular, pain specialists and organizations were calling for a treatment model similar to the one developed by the World Health Organization (WHO) in 1986 (Fig. 1.2): the "analgesic ladder for managing cancer pain" encouraged physicians to take a stepwise approach to managing cancer pain by starting with nonopioid analgesics before advancing to "weak" and then "stronger" opioids. This pharmacologic guide served not only to sanction the use of opioids for end-of-life cancer pain, but it also reignited the debate about how

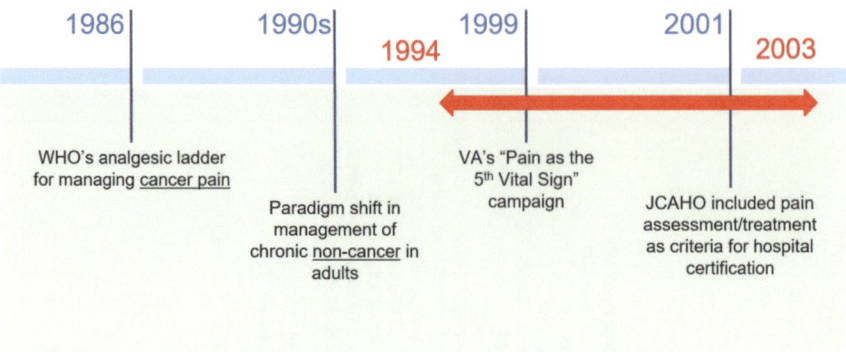

Fig. 1.2 Roots of the opioid crisis. This figure shows the timeline for the major events that played a role in the opioid epidemic

to care for patients who suffered chronically from pain that was not due to cancer. One of the most prominent advocates for using opioids to treat chronic noncancer pain was Russell Portenoy, a pain specialist in New York and professor of neurology and neuroscience, who argued that the medical establishment had failed to address chronic pain and had ignored the suffering of millions of Americans [12].

1.5 "Pain as the 5th Vital Sign"

The view that pain was being undertreated in the United States was reflected in a keynote address delivered on November 11, 1995, by Dr. Joseph Campbell, who was then head of the American Pain Society. In his presidential address, Dr. Campbell introduced the term *pain as the 5th vital sign* [13, 14]. With these six words, Dr. Campbell set in motion a fundamental shift in how we treat and manage pain in this country and, some argue, laid the groundwork for the largest drug crisis in this country's history.

> "Vital signs are taken seriously. If pain were assessed with the same zeal as other vital signs are, it would have a much better chance of being treated properly. We need to train doctors and nurses to treat pain as a vital sign. Quality care means that pain is measured and treated," stated Dr. Campbell.

This was a seminal event, and within a few years, two key stakeholders adopted the use of "pain as the 5th vital sign" metric. In 1996, the Department of Veterans Affairs included the metric as part of its national pain management strategy, and in 1998, the Joint Commission on Accreditation of Hospital Organizations (JCAHO) adopted it as part of their criteria for hospital evaluation. Yet, the standards of care adopted by JCAHO never mention drugs in general, or opioids specifically, for the treatment of pain. It only states that pain should be assessed in all patients. However, in 2000, JCAHO published a book that was marketed to physicians citing that "there is no evidence that addiction is a serious issue when opioids are given for pain control" [14]. The book also stated that concerns about opioid addiction were inaccurate and exaggerated.

The book was sponsored by Purdue Pharma—one of only two drug companies that provided funding for JCAHO's educational programs related to pain management [15]. Furthermore, in an agreement between Purdue Pharma and JCAHO, Purdue was the *only* drug company allowed to distribute a book related to pain management and certain educational videos [16]. JCAHO made these materials available for purchase on its website. According to the United States Government Accountability Office, the partnership between the JCAHO and Purdue may have helped the drug company gain access to hospitals to further the promotion of OxyContin [15].

Despite these sweeping changes in pain assessment and management philosophy, healthcare systems consistently failed to implement safety measures that should have accompanied such a dramatic shift in practice. In my research examining guideline-concordant care for US veterans receiving opioids for chronic pain between 1998 and 2010, I found that despite mounting evidence of risk and increasingly detailed clinical practice guidelines, healthcare systems continued to struggle with implementing basic safety measures [17]. Over this decade, patients received no more than 40% of recommended monitoring and safety assessments—a failure that persisted even as evidence of opioid-related harms mounted. This implementation gap is particularly striking given that the VA healthcare system, which championed the "pain as the 5th vital sign" initiative, should have been better positioned than most healthcare systems to implement comprehensive safety measures. It was in this context of rapid change in prescribing practices without corresponding safety protocols that Purdue Pharma introduced OxyContin, a high-dose and extended-release version of oxycodone that would fundamentally transform the treatment of pain in America [15].

1.6   OxyContin: A New Drug, a Deadly Crisis

OxyContin was introduced in the midst of this cultural zeitgeist. By the time the Food and Drug Administration (FDA) approved the "new drug" in 1996 for the treatment of "moderate-to-severe pain lasting more than a few days," the paradigm shift sought by Purdue Pharma in the way doctors perceived of opioids and pain treatment was well underway [12]. The groundwork had been laid for Purdue to launch one of the most aggressive and successful drug marketing campaigns ever seen to promote OxyContin.

Between 1996 and 2001, according to a congressional report prepared by the United States Government Accountability Office, Purdue carried out at least 40 national conferences that focused on pain management and in training spokespeople for its National Speaker's Bureau [15]. These symposia were held in glamorous resorts, such as Boca Raton, Florida, and Scottsdale, Arizona, and attended by physicians, specialists in pain medicine, nurses, and pharmacists who had been recruited by Purdue Pharma—who covered all costs of travel, lodging, and meals for more than 5000 attendees in total [15]. The overarching goal was to educate healthcare providers on the appropriate use of opioids, including OxyContin, so that they in turn could reach their colleagues in various medical settings, such as local conferences and grand round presentations—which are attended by physicians, residents, and medical trainees. Sales representatives from Purdue also attended these conferences with the aim of influencing physician prescribing practices [15]. Sales representatives, in addition to a base salary of approximately $50,000, would receive bonuses based on the number of prescriptions written for OxyContin in their territories. These bonuses ranged from $15,000 to $240,000 annually [18]. In 2001 alone, Purdue paid $40 million in incentives to sales representatives [18].

By way of example, as part of this campaign, in 1998, Purdue created and distributed 15,000 copies of a video intended for physician waiting rooms. "I Got My Life Back" chronicled the stories of six patients with chronic pain who were treated with OxyContin [15]. A doctor tells of how these patients were able to go on working and living their lives without pain or serious side effects. According to Purdue, OxyContin would provide patients with 12 h of continuous pain relief, all in a form that was nonaddictive owing to its controlled-release properties [15]. Purdue did not submit the video to the FDA for review as stipulated by regulations that govern the oversight of promotional activities [18].

Within a year of the video's release, opioid prescriptions rose by 11 million, and by 1999, sales of OxyContin were generating $20 million per week [12]. In total, between 1996 and 2002, Purdue funded more than 20,000 educational programs related to pain management through financial grants or direct sponsorship—all with the intent of influencing physician prescribing practices [18].

Among the most questionable practices Purdue engaged in was to distribute coupons to physicians who were then to give them to patients who could present the coupons at pharmacies for a one-time supply (between 7 and 30 days) of OxyContin at no cost [18]. The program ran intermittently for 4 years. In 2001, when the program ended, 34,000 coupons had been redeemed by patients [15].

With the help of physicians, most of whom were well-meaning, and leading healthcare organizations, such as the Department of Veterans Affairs, Purdue had achieved with its aggressive marketing plan what they set out to do. All told, the marketing of OxyContin catapulted retail sales of the drug. In 1996, there were approximately 316,000 OxyContin prescriptions dispensed, amounting to $48 million in sales. By 2001, OxyContin had become the most prescribed name-brand opioid for treating moderate to severe pain in the United States [18]. Combined sales in 2001 and 2002 reveal that the number of OxyContin prescriptions dispensed exceeded 14 million and sales reached nearly $3 billion [18]. The majority of these prescriptions were for noncancerous conditions. Whereas OxyContin prescriptions for cancer pain increased approximately fourfold between 1997 and 2002, prescriptions of the drug for noncancer pain increased nearly tenfold [15, 18].

Purdue used its influence on primary care physicians to promote OxyContin as an initial opioid treatment for noncancerous conditions. By 2003, nearly half of those prescribing the drug were primary care doctors, many of whom were not adequately trained in pain management. Experts at the time, including members of the US Drug Enforcement Agency, were concerned about the lack of training and the amount of time available for primary care doctors for adequately evaluating the risks and benefits of treatment and sufficiently following up with patients suffering from chronic pain to ensure that they were not experiencing adverse effects, including dependency or signs of addiction [18].

In 2009, the *American Journal of Public Health* published an in-depth analysis of Purdue Pharma's promotion and of marketing OxyContin and the events that followed [18]. This analysis was written by Dr. Art Van Zee, a primary care physician who practices in St. Charles, Virginia, a small coal mining town in Southwest Virginia, an area of the country hit particularly hard by the opioid crisis [18]. As summed up by Van Zee, "OxyContin's commercial success did not depend upon the merits of the drug compared to other available opioid preparations." The medical review officer at the FDA, in evaluating Purdue's new application, concluded that OxyContin (extended release) did not offer a significant advantage over its predecessor—oxycodone (immediate release), except in terms of the frequency of dosing [18]. Randomized, double-blind clinical trials conducted within 5 years of OxyContin hitting the market bore this out. OxyContin taken on a 12-h schedule was comparable to oxycodone taken on a 4-h schedule in terms of efficacy (the capacity of a drug to produce the desired effect) and safety in either patients with chronic back pain or those suffering from cancer pain.

In 2007, criminal charges were brought against an affiliate of Purdue Pharma, Purdue Frederick Company, for claiming that OxyContin was less addictive and less prone to abuse and diversion for nonmedical use (e.g., selling the drug to someone for recreational purposes). Three executives pled guilty. The makers of OxyContin had claimed from the beginning that the drug was less prone to abuse than other opioids such as oxycodone because of its controlled-release formulation. At the time OxyContin was approved in 1996, the FDA also believed that because the drug would be absorbed slowly, it would not offer a rush or a high, and according to the FDA's website [19] that presents a timeline of significant events related to the opioid epidemic, there was no evidence at the time that crushing the controlled-release tablet in order to ingest or snort the contents would be a widespread practice and lead to significant levels of abuse. But in fact, according to Dr. Van Zee, "Purdue knew from its own test in 1995 that 68% of oxycodone could be extracted from the tablet when crushed." It is unclear whether these data were included in the initial drug application to the FDA. Purdue had gone to great effort to minimize the risks of addiction for those being treated for noncancer pain. One promotional video that Purdue distributed to physicians claimed that OxyContin resulted in addiction in less than half of 1% of these patients [18].

Because of Purdue's promotion of OxyContin specifically and opioids in general, not only did OxyContin sales increase exponentially, but the sales of other opioids did as well [15]. Purdue had set in motion the largest drug crisis the world had ever seen—one we are still living with today.

References

1. Drug Enforcement Agency. Opium Poppy. https://museum.dea.gov/exhibits/online-exhibits/cannabis-coca-and-poppy-natures-addictive-plants/opium-poppy. Accessed 14 June 2024.
2. Schmitt, K. A brief history of opioids in the U.S. 2023. https://magazine.publichealth.jhu.edu/2023/brief-history-opioids-us. Accessed 14 June 2024.
3. Krishnamurti C, Rao SC. The isolation of morphine by Serturner. Indian J Anaesth. 2016;60(11):861–2. https://doi.org/10.4103/0019-5049.193696.
4. Batmanabane G. Why patients in pain cannot get "God's own medicine?". J Pharmacol Pharmacother. 2014;5(2):81–2. https://doi.org/10.4103/0976-500X.130040.
5. Macy B. Dopesick: dealers, doctors, and the drug company that addicted America. 1st ed. New York: Little, Brown and Company; 2018.
6. Adams JFA. Substitutes for opium in chronic diseases. Boston Med Surg J. 1888;121:351.
7. Porter J, Jick H. Addiction rare in patients treated with narcotics. N Engl J Med. 1980;302(2):123. https://doi.org/10.1056/nejm198001103020221.
8. Leung PTM, Macdonald EM, Stanbrook MB, Dhalla IA, Juurlink DN. A 1980 letter on the risk of opioid addiction. N Engl J Med. 2017;376(22):2194–5. https://doi.org/10.1056/NEJMc1700150.
9. Miller FG, Joffe S. Equipoise and the dilemma of randomized clinical trials. N Engl J Med. 2011;364(5):476–80. https://doi.org/10.1056/NEJMsb1011301.
10. Kowal N. What is the issue? Pseudoaddiction or undertreatment of pain. Nurs Econ. 1999;17(6):348–9.
11. Ronald TL, Coherent D. Treating doctors as drug dealers: the DEA's war on prescription painkillers. Washington, DC: Policy Analysis. Cato Institute; 2005.
12. Keefe PR. Empire of pain: the secret history of the Sackler dynasty. New York: Doubleday; 2021.
13. Humble W. The 5th vital sign: the painkiller epidemic part I of V. 2014. https://directorsblog.health.azdhs.gov/the-5th-vital-sign-the-painkiller-epidemic-part-i-of-v/. Accessed 14 June 2024.
14. Mandell BF. The fifth vital sign: a complex story of politics and patient care. Cleve Clin J Med. 2016;83(6):400–1. https://doi.org/10.3949/ccjm.83b.06016.
15. U.S. Government Accounting Office. Prescription drugs: oxycontin abuse and diversion and efforts to address the problem. GAO-04-110. 2003.
16. Chhabra N, Leikin JB. The joint commission and the opioid epidemic. JAMA. 2017;318(1):91–2. https://doi.org/10.1001/jama.2017.6694.
17. Gaither JR, Goulet JL, Becker WC, et al. The association between receipt of guideline-concordant long-term opioid therapy and all-cause mortality. J Gen Intern Med. 2016;31(5):492–501. https://doi.org/10.1007/s11606-015-3571-4.
18. Van Zee A. The promotion and marketing of oxycontin: commercial triumph, public health tragedy. Am J Public Health. 2009;99(2):221–7. https://doi.org/10.2105/AJPH.2007.131714.
19. Food and Drug Administration. Timeline of selected FDA activities and significant events addressing substance use and overdose prevention. https://www.fda.gov/drugs/food-and-drug-administration-overdose-prevention-framework/timeline-selected-fda-activities-and-significant-events-addressing-substance-use-and-overdose. Accessed 18 Jan 2025.

The US Opioid Epidemic: An Evolving and Systemic Crisis

2

The US opioid epidemic represents one of the most catastrophic public health crises in recent history, evolving over three decades and distinct waves. This chapter examines how what began as a prescription drug crisis—driven largely by the aggressive marketing of OxyContin—transformed into an epidemic of heroin use and ultimately a crisis dominated by illegally manufactured fentanyl. The geographic progression of the epidemic from rural Appalachia to a nationwide crisis is mapped alongside changing demographic patterns that have increasingly affected minority populations and women. By analyzing prescribing patterns, overdose rates, and policy responses, this chapter reveals how attempts to address one aspect of the crisis often led to an inadvertent worsening of other aspects. The devastating impact of the epidemic is quantified not only in terms of mortality—with recent data showing approximately 200 deaths per day from fentanyl alone—but also through its profound effects on communities, healthcare systems, and vulnerable populations, including women and children.

2.1 The Aftermath of OxyContin: From Regional Hot Spots to National Crisis

The commercial success of OxyContin was unprecedented, as was the devastation it caused to communities across the United States. "We know of no other medication routinely used for a nonfatal condition that kills patients so frequently," stated Dr. Tom Frieden, former Director of the Centers for Disease Control and Prevention (CDC), in 2016 [1].

In 2009, the *American Journal of Public Health* published an in-depth analysis of Purdue Pharma's promotion and of marketing OxyContin and the events that followed. This analysis was written by Dr. Van Zee, the primary care physician introduced in Chap. 1, who practices in the small coal mining town in Southwest Virginia [2]. As outlined in his analysis, reports of the abuse and diversion of OxyContin began to emerge around 1999 and 2000 in several geographic hot spots, including in Alabama, eastern Kentucky, Maine, and West Virginia. In each of these areas, the rates at which OxyContin was prescribed were notably higher than the national average—up to five to six times higher in some areas. For example, in 2000, nationally, there were 3750 grams of OxyContin distributed per 100,000 population, but in Dickenson, Virginia, the region with the highest prescribing rate, there were nearly 26,000 grams distributed per 100,000. But it was not only OxyContin that was being prescribed well above the national average in certain areas. Other opioids, such as hydrocodone and oxycodone (non-OxyContin), were being prescribed excessively as well.

As the number of opioid prescriptions rose, so did rates of abuse and admissions to opioid treatment facilities (e.g., methadone maintenance programs), diversion of opioids for nonmedical use, and overdose deaths. Between 1997 and 2003, deaths from prescription opioids rose 834% in southwest Virginia. Within 3 years after the first methadone maintenance treatment (MMT) program opened in this region in 2000, there had been 1400 admissions. A similar pattern emerged in other areas, which were mostly rural. In response to the growing number of individuals dependent upon OxyContin, West Virginia also opened its first MMT program in 2000. By 2023, there were seven such programs in the state, treating more than 3000 patients. Eastern Kentucky saw a 500% increase in the number of patients admitted to MMT programs between 1995 and 2001, with approximately three-quarters of patients dependent on OxyContin [2].

Most of these five regions are rural and all except Maine are part of Appalachia. Dr. Zee does not address in depth the reasons why opioid prescribing rates were the highest in these areas. Historically in this country, drug epidemics have started in urban areas before spreading to rural communities. Why was this epidemic different? In his article published in 2009, he states only that "The regions of the country that had the earliest and highest availability of prescribed OxyContin had the greatest initial abuse and diversion." It all came down to the availability of OxyContin in these regions [2].

Within just a few years, Appalachia's regional problem with opioids in general—and OxyContin in particular—soon became a national problem. The rising tide of abuse, diversion, and overdose spread from rural areas of the country to large cities as well as suburban communities. No region of the country was spared. Nationally, between 1997 and 2002, prescriptions for all opioids increased dramatically. Morphine and fentanyl prescriptions increased 226% and 73%, respectively. By far, though, the largest increase in opioid prescribing was for oxycodone, and nearly three-quarters of these prescriptions were for OxyContin. By 2004, OxyContin had become the most abused opioid in the country. According to the Substance Abuse and Mental Health Services Administration (SAMHSA), among those who were considered new initiates to illicit drug use in 2005—2.1 million people—the first drugs they tried were prescription opioids [2, 3]. This surpassed the number reporting that the first drug they tried was marijuana, and it was nearly equal to the number reported for cigarette use: 2.3 million.

Consistent with the pattern seen in rural areas, the dramatic increase in the availability of opioids, including OxyContin, was correlated with rising rates of abuse, diversion, and death. National data show that by the early 2000s, accidental overdose deaths from prescription opioids surpassed deaths from heroin and cocaine as well as from firearm injuries and motor vehicle accidents.

2.2 Rising Availability and Deaths: The First Wave

National data show that in 1997, on average, healthcare providers wrote 59 outpatient opioid prescriptions for every 100 US residents. By 2018, 51 opioid prescriptions were prescribed for every 100 people, which still represents annual prescriptions in excess of 168 million. The latest data from the CDC shows that in 2023, there were 38 prescriptions dispensed per 100 people in the United States. But in Arkansas, Alabama, and Mississippi, rates are more than double the national average.

In 1999, according to the CDC, the amounts of opioids prescribed as measured in milligrams of morphine equivalents (MMEs) were 180 per person in the United States [4] (milligrams of morphine equivalents is a measure that quantifies the potency of an opioid relative to morphine, the first modern opioid used for pain treatment). By 2015, the per person MME was 640. Between 1999 and 2010, there were enough opioids prescribed to "medicate every American adult with a standard pain treatment dose of 5 mg of hydrocode (Vicodin and others) taken every 4 hours for a month" [5].

When considering these statistics, it is important to note that they tell only part of the story. Not only did the number of prescriptions dispensed increase, but because of the shift in the use of opioids for managing chronic pain (as opposed to treating pain associated with acute injuries or end-of-life), the amount of opioids prescribed also increased, as did the dosages required to overcome the tolerance patients built up to the drugs over time [4]. All of which meant that more patients were prescribed opioids at ever-increasing dosages and for longer periods of time. In the decade between 1997 and 2007, average sales in grams of opioids prescribed per person increased from 74 to 369 mg—an increase of 402% [6] (Fig. 2.1).

But higher prescribing in terms of the number of prescriptions, higher doses, and length of time did not equate to higher safety. With rising sales came a parallel rise in overdose deaths due to opioids. From 1997 to 2007, opioid sales increased nearly sixfold, and with each year, deaths attributed to opioid overdoses rose in tandem. In just over a decade, between 1997 and 2008, the rate of drug overdoses from prescription opioids increased by nearly 400%. In 2008 alone, prescription opioids were implicated in the deaths of nearly 15,000 people across the country. Nearly 100 people a day were dying from drug overdoses, approximately three-quarters of which were caused by prescription opioids. But fatality rates varied widely across the United States. The CDC's assessment of the underlying forces behind this variability is in line with the conclusions drawn by Dr. Zee: "Wide variation among states in the nonmedical use of OPR [opioid pain relievers] and overdose rates cannot be explained by underlying demographic differences in state populations but is related to wide variations in OPR prescribing" [2].

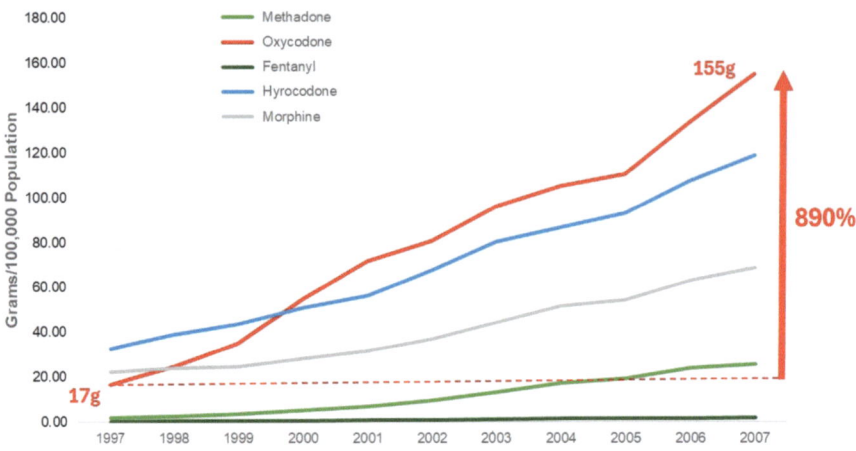

Fig. 2.1 Therapeutic use of opioids in the United States (mg/person), 1997–2007. Average sales in grams prescribed per person in the United States between 1997 and 2007. (Source: US Drug Enforcement Administration. Adapted from Manchikanti et al. [6])

But it is also true that many of the patients who were prescribed opioids were predominately white men from rural areas, many of whom were already vulnerable and at high risk because of poverty, chronic illness, or a history of mental health or substance use disorders. Patients with a history of depression were more likely to receive a higher daily dose of opioids, more Schedule II opioids (opioids with a high potential for abuse), and a larger days' supply. Duration of use is known to be the strongest predictor for addiction and overdose. For each additional week that a patient stays on a prescribed opioid, the risk associated with opioid use disorder (OUD) and overdose increase by 20% [7–9].

2.3 Unintended Consequences: The Reformulation of OxyContin

In 2010, OxyContin, which was originally developed to be taken whole, was reformulated with a polyethylene oxide coating that served to harden the tablets so that the contents could not be aspirated and subsequently injected. The new abuse-deterrent formulation put in place mechanical barriers that also made it resistant to crushing, chewing, and snorting. In August of that year, shipments of the original formulation ceased, and the new formulation was made commercially available. By December 2010, 90% of OxyContin prescriptions dispensed were for the reformulated version of OxyContin [10]. The FDA allowed Purdue Pharma to change the drug label for OxyContin to emphasize the abuse-deterrent properties of the reformulated version [11].

According to a study by Thomas Cicero from the Department of Psychiatry at Washington University, the reformulation did have an immediate impact on the abuse of the drug, but it was short-lived, and any public health gains in terms of stemming abuse of the drug eventually leveled out. In interviews that the researchers conducted among a sample of individuals with a history of abusing OxyContin, approximately one-third said that they persisted in abusing OxyContin; they simply stopped injecting or inhaling the drug and started taking it orally, whereas others found a way to get around the abuse-deterrent barriers and continued to snort or inject the contents [11].

Although there was an immediate drop in rates for abusing the drug, according to a recent analysis by Beachler et al., there was "little or no change" in overdose rates for OxyContin following the reformulation among insured patients receiving routine medical care [10].

2.4 The Second Wave: Heroin Fills the Prescription Void

Overall, in defiance of expectations among those who had for years called for Purdue Pharma to reformulate the drug, doing so only made things worse [12] and ushered in the second wave of the opioid crisis: the illicit opioid phase. The barriers to misusing the prescription form of OxyContin drove many people to abuse other opioids, including those found on the black market. Overwhelmingly, patients turned to heroin—a drug that was both easier to obtain than OxyContin and cheaper to purchase. As illustrated by quotes from the Cicero study noted above, many patients saw the move from using prescription opioids to heroin as the most practical and economically smart alternative. As one participant in the study said: "…I heard heroin would get me higher and was cheaper, and when Oxys changed, so did my choice of drug" [11].

Prior to 2010, the predominant supplier of heroin in the United States was South America, but coinciding with the increased demand for an alternative to OxyContin, Mexico stepped in to become the predominant producer of the drug, ensuring a reliable supply at a low cost. Cicero and colleagues found that the drug of choice for those switching from OxyContin was heroin; more than 70% of study participants, in fact, switched to heroin [11]. In general, a 40-mg tablet of OxyContin is sold on the street for roughly $40 and an 80-mg tablet for $80, so roughly $1 per milligram. In contrast, a single-dose bag of heroin could be purchased for between $5 and $20.

As Malcolm Gladwell points out in his book *Revenge of the Tipping Point*, which includes an insightful analysis of the opioid epidemic from a lay person [12]:

> As strange as it is to say this, if you must have an opioid epidemic, these are the group proportions you want: You want the majority of users to be dependent on prescription drugs. A prescription-drug epidemic is powered by a company operating within the law, answerable to shareholders, and regulated by a government agency. The prescribers are medical professionals. Every transaction between company and physician, and every transaction between physician and patient, is recorded. Insurers—public and private—reimburse users. When things go wrong, we know they are going wrong. We have levers to push. We can find the superspreader doctors and try to stop them, track their patients and try to help them.

The Cicero study highlights the extent to which the vast majority of OxyContin abusers, including those who received their opioids through prescription, were willing to endure the stigma associated with heroin in order to stave off withdrawing from opioids [11]. Cicero concludes this study by stating that supply-side interventions, such as reformulating OxyContin to deter abuse, are insufficient to address the opioid crisis and that more comprehensive solutions are needed.

From a public health perspective, the transition from prescribed opioids to heroin was disastrous given the lethality of heroin, which is two to three times stronger than morphine. Heroin use exposes individuals not only to a higher overdose risk, but also to the risks associated with drug injections, such as HIV and crime [11].

As heroin deaths began to rise, those from commonly prescribed opioids, including OxyContin, began leveling off. By 2015, annual deaths from heroin surpassed those from prescription opioids [13]. Between 2010 and 2017, overdose deaths from heroin increased by approximately 400%, whereas deaths from prescription opioids rose less than 100% [13]. In 2010, nationwide there were 3036 deaths from heroin; by 2016, there were 15,469 [14]. Since 2016, heroin overdose deaths have been trending down, but in 2022, there were approximately 6000 deaths per year from the drug.

2.5 Fentanyl: The Third and Deadliest Wave

Unfortunately, heroin ushered in a rise in deaths from other illicit drugs, including fentanyl, which marked the beginning of the third, and deadliest, wave of the opioid epidemic. Beginning around 2013, the United States was flooded with fentanyl, a drug that historically had been prescribed for severe pain, such as post-operative pain. Fentanyl, a synthetic opioid, as opposed to a natural opioid that is derived from the poppy plant, is considered 50 times more potent than heroin and 100 times more potent than morphine.

Pharmaceutical-grade fentanyl was developed in 1959 by Dr. Paul Janssen, a Belgian physician and founder of Janssen Pharmaceutica, now a subsidiary of Johnson & Johnson [15]. The Food and Drug Administration approved fentanyl as a pain reliever and anesthetic in 1968 [16]. The agent was first introduced to the market as an intravenous anesthetic branded Sublimaze [15]. Up until the 1990s, the use of fentanyl was largely confined to the operating room, but with the development of the fentanyl patch in the 1990s, the medication could be delivered transdermally. With the Duragesic patch, as it was branded, a steady dose of fentanyl could be delivered throughout the day to patients suffering from chronic pain.

Because fentanyl is a synthetic opioid, meaning that it is created in a lab, it could be manufactured illegally. And it was illegally manufactured fentanyl (IMF) that started the latest, but likely not the last, wave of the opioid epidemic. Fentanyl as a prescription medication continues to be legally manufactured and distributed in the United States, and as with any prescription opioid, it is frequently diverted for illicit use through illegal channels. But much of the fentanyl that makes its way to the market is illegally manufactured in labs outside of the United States—primarily Mexico and China.

Beginning in the early 2000s, there were reports of fentanyl overdoses in localized areas of the country. Nationwide the number of deaths attributed to synthetic opioids was in the range of 700 per year. But in 2013, there was a sharp rise in deaths from fentanyl. In that year, there were approximately 3000 deaths across the United States attributed to fentanyl, which correlated highly with an unprecedented rise in the production and distribution of IMF, fueled by an increase in the global supply of fentanyl chemicals produced by criminal organizations. There was no correlation with an increase in fentanyl prescribing rates. Between 2013 and 2014, the number of drugs seized by law enforcement that tested positive for fentanyl increased by 426%. In 2015, the Drug Enforcement Administration (DEA) and CDC issued nationwide alerts identifying IMFs as a threat to public health and safety [17]. These alerts had little impact, though. By 2016, deaths from fentanyl had surpassed deaths from heroin, and by 2017, the number of fentanyl deaths had surpassed 28,000. Deaths from fentanyl now account for approximately 70,000 a year—100 times the number of deaths reported in 2000.

Fentanyl is now the primary driver of the opioid crisis and in 2023 was responsible for 92% of opioid-related overdoses, according to the most up-to-date CDC data [18, 19]. Approximately 200 people die in this country every day from a fentanyl overdose [14, 18]. Over the past 5 years, more than 300,000 Americans have lost their lives to the drug [20].

The proliferation of IMF, which primarily enters the United States through major ports of entry, has led to dramatic demographic changes since 2013 in the groups vulnerable to opioid fatalities. IMF and its derivatives, which are often found in other illicit drugs, such as cocaine, counterfeit prescription pills, and methamphetamine, have meant that Black people are now disproportionately represented in overdose fatalities. In fact, nearly every racial and ethnic group has seen a significant rise in opioid overdoses in the past decade [20].

2.6 Changing Demographics: From White Men to Minorities, Women, and Children

When you look closely at the data, you see clearly how the opioid epidemic as it relates to opioids in general and fentanyl specifically has evolved not only as it relates to implicated drugs (prescription opioids, heroin, and fentanyl) but also in terms of location, race, and, most troublingly, age.

Initially, deaths from fentanyl were largely confined to eight states, seven of which were located in the Northeast (Massachusetts, Maine, and New Hampshire) or the South (Florida, Kentucky, Maryland, and North Carolina). Only one state in the Midwest, Ohio, had significant deaths from IMFs. Currently, West Virginia has the highest fentanyl overdose rate of any state at 67 deaths per 100,000 residents, which is significantly higher than the rates in South Dakota, the least affected state, where fentanyl overdose rates are estimated at 4.6 per 100,000 residents [21]. In fact, fentanyl in 2021 was the leading cause of drug overdose deaths in all regions of the country. In total, more than a quarter million have died nationwide from fentanyl since 2018.

The evolution we see in terms of location can also be seen in regard to race/ethnicity and age. In the early stages of the opioid crisis, the epidemic of drug use and overdose was largely confined to young and middle-aged white males. Historically, minority populations have had low rates of opioid overdose. But with each successive wave of the opioid epidemic, the impact has spread to all sectors of society—including women, children, and minorities. In 2010, for example, whites had the highest overdose rates. By 2020, rates were the highest among Blacks. The reasons for this are complex but rooted in part in prescribing practices for Black patients [22], who, during the prescription opioid wave, were less likely than white patients to be prescribed an opioid for chronic pain—or if they did receive a prescription, the strength of the drug was lower than would be given to a white patient with comparable pain. Research suggests that these practices, which point to structural racism within the healthcare system, likely had a protective effect early in the epidemic. But the lack of access to prescription opioids over time has caused many Black patients to turn to street drugs.

2.7 Social Determinants and Vulnerable Populations

The differential impact of the opioid epidemic across demographic groups illustrates how social determinants of health profoundly influence addiction vulnerability and treatment outcomes. Economic factors have played a critical role, with the epidemic's earliest waves disproportionately affecting communities suffering from limited economic opportunities due to deindustrialization and declining coal and manufacturing industries. Educational attainment, housing instability, and healthcare access have emerged as crucial factors for determining the vulnerability of communities to opioids, as have social isolation and the erosion of support systems in areas with population decline. These socioeconomic factors intersect with racial disparities in healthcare [22], creating complex patterns of vulnerability that have evolved across the epidemic's three waves (Fig. 2.2).

Among the most concerning of these demographic shifts has been the increased use of opioids among women. Between 1999 and 2017, fatal overdoses increased by nearly 500% among women 30–64 years of age. Research shows that women are prescribed opioids in greater numbers than men and are also more likely than men to develop an opioid use disorder [23]. There are several factors that make women particularly vulnerable to opioids. Smaller body mass index, metabolism, and tolerance can make opioids more addictive and lethal for women [24]. The growing public health crisis among women during the transition from the first to the second wave of the opioid epidemic has only served to heighten the risks that opioids pose to women, including women of reproductive age, with particularly

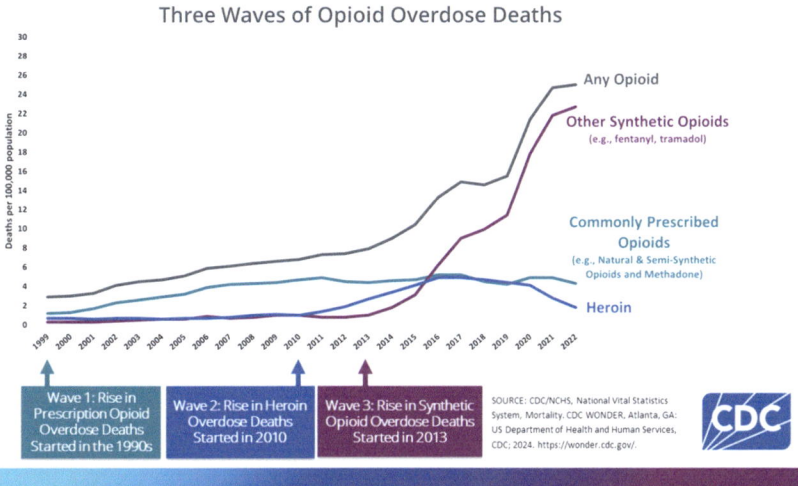

Fig. 2.2 The Three Waves of the Opioid Epidemic. This figure illustrates the three distinct waves of the opioid epidemic and how opioid overdose deaths have increased over the past three decades

devastating consequences for pregnant women and newborns—a topic we will explore in the next chapter.

References

1. Frieden TR, Houry D. Reducing the risks of relief--the CDC opioid-prescribing guideline. N Engl J Med. 2016;374(16):1501–4. https://doi.org/10.1056/NEJMp1515917.
2. Van Zee A. The promotion and marketing of oxycontin: commercial triumph, public health tragedy. Am J Public Health. 2009;99(2):221–7. https://doi.org/10.2105/AJPH.2007.131714.
3. Substance Abuse and Mental Health Services Administration. National survey on drug use and health. https://www.samhsa.gov/data/data-we-collect/nsduh-national-survey-drug-use-and-health/national-releases/older. Accessed 18 Jan 2025.
4. Guy GP Jr, Zhang K, Bohm MK, et al. Vital signs: changes in opioid prescribing in the United States, 2006–2015. MMWR Morb Mortal Wkly Rep. 2017;66(26):697–704. https://doi.org/10.15585/mmwr.mm6626a4.
5. Centers for Disease Control and Prevention. Vital signs: overdoses of prescription opioid pain relievers–United States, 1999–2008. MMWR Morb Mortal Wkly Rep. 2011;60(43):1487–92.
6. Manchikanti L, Fellows B, Ailinani H, Pampati V. Therapeutic use, abuse, and nonmedical use of opioids: a ten-year perspective. Pain Physician. 2010;13(5):401–35.
7. Schieber LZ, Guy GP Jr, Seth P, et al. Trends and patterns of geographic variation in opioid prescribing practices by state, United States, 2006–2017. JAMA Netw Open. 2019;2(3):e190665. https://doi.org/10.1001/jamanetworkopen.2019.0665.
8. Edlund MJ, Austen MA, Sullivan MD, et al. Patterns of opioid use for chronic noncancer pain in the Veterans Health Administration from 2009 to 2011. Pain. 2014;155(11):2337–43. https://doi.org/10.1016/j.pain.2014.08.033.

9. Brat GA, Agniel D, Beam A, et al. Postsurgical prescriptions for opioid naive patients and association with overdose and misuse: retrospective cohort study. BMJ. 2018;360:j5790. https://doi.org/10.1136/bmj.j5790.
10. Beachler DC, Hall K, Garg R, et al. An evaluation of the effect of the OxyContin reformulation on unintentional fatal and nonfatal overdose. Clin J Pain. 2022;38(6):396–404. https://doi.org/10.1097/AJP.0000000000001034.
11. Cicero TJ, Ellis MS. Abuse-deterrent formulations and the prescription opioid abuse epidemic in the United States: lessons learned from OxyContin. JAMA Psychiatry. 2015;72(5):424–30. https://doi.org/10.1001/jamapsychiatry.2014.3043.
12. Gladwell M. Revenge of the tipping point: overstories, superspreaders and the rise of social engineering. Abacus Books; 2024.
13. Ciccarone D. The triple wave epidemic: supply and demand drivers of the US opioid overdose crisis. Int J Drug Policy. 2019;71:183–8. https://doi.org/10.1016/j.drugpo.2019.01.010.
14. National Institute on Drug Abuse. Drug overdose deaths: facts and figures. https://nida.nih.gov/research-topics/trends-statistics/overdose-death-rates#:~:text=U.S.%20Overdose%20Deaths%20Involving%20Heroin,Other%20Opioid%20Involvement%2C%201999%2D2022&text=Drug%20overdose%20deaths%20involving%20heroin,5%2C871%20reported%20deaths%20in%202022. Accessed 1 Feb 2025.
15. Stanley TH. The fentanyl story. J Pain. 2014;15(12):1215–26. https://doi.org/10.1016/j.jpain.2014.08.010.
16. Food and Drug Administration. Timeline of selected FDA activities and significant events addressing substance use and overdose prevention. https://www.fda.gov/drugs/food-and-drug-administration-overdose-prevention-framework/timeline-selected-fda-activities-and-significant-events-addressing-substance-use-and-overdose. Accessed 18 Jan 2025.
17. Gladden RM, Martinez P, Seth P. Fentanyl law enforcement submissions and increases in synthetic opioid-involved overdose deaths – 27 states, 2013–2014. MMWR Morb Mortal Wkly Rep. 2016;65(33):837–43. https://doi.org/10.15585/mmwr.mm6533a2.
18. Centers for Disease Control and Prevention. About overdose prevention. https://www.cdc.gov/overdose-prevention/about/index.html. Accessed 14 Aug 2025.
19. Gaither JR. National trends in pediatric deaths from fentanyl, 1999–2021. JAMA Pediatr. 2023. https://doi.org/10.1001/jamapediatrics.2023.0793.
20. Spencer MR, Garnett M, Miniño AM, National Center for Health Statistics. Drug overdose deaths in the United States, 2002–2022. NCHS data brief no 491. U.S. Department of Health and Human Services, Centers for Disease Control and Prevention, National Center for Health Statistics; 2024.
21. USAFacts. Who is overdosing on fentanyl? https://usafacts.org/articles/who-is-overdosing-on-fentanyl/. Accessed 14 Aug 2025.
22. Gaither JR, Gordon K, Crystal S, et al. Racial disparities in discontinuation of long-term opioid therapy following illicit drug use among black and white patients. Drug Alcohol Depend. 2018;192:371–6. https://doi.org/10.1016/j.drugalcdep.2018.05.033.
23. Springer SA, Biondi BE, Frank C, El-Bassel N. A call to action to combat the opioid epidemic among women. J Addict Med. 2020;14(5):364–6. https://doi.org/10.1097/ADM.0000000000000622.
24. Gaither JR. The impact of the opioid crisis on neonates, children, and adolescents. In: Suresh S, Shah R, editors. Opioid therapy in children and adolescents. 1st ed. Springer Science; 2020. p. 17–30.

3

Neonatal Opioid Withdrawal Syndrome: Clinical Challenges and Evolving Approaches to Care

The maternal opioid epidemic has led to a substantial increase in the number of infants born with neonatal opioid withdrawal syndrome (NOWS). This chapter examines the immediate and long-term challenges faced by these infants and their families. Infants with NOWS present with a distinctive constellation of symptoms, including nervous system irritability, autonomic nervous system overactivity, and gastrointestinal dysregulation, resulting in an extended length of stay for the newborn hospitalization. The financial burden of caring for infants with NOWS has placed substantial strain on the US healthcare system, with annual costs escalating over the past two decades from tens of millions to more than half a billion dollars. These economic pressures, combined with clinical concerns about the treatment of infants and families affected by maternal opioid use, have driven recent innovation in the field. This chapter examines the evolution from the traditional Finnegan approach to the newer Eat, Sleep, Console (ESC) model, which emphasizes family-centered care. Beyond the immediate postpartum period, research indicates that infants with NOWS face elevated risks for hospital readmission, particularly for neglect, failure to thrive, and traumatic injuries. The chapter concludes with recommendations for improved discharge planning, highlighting the need for standardized and integrated care models that address both the infant's medical needs and the mother's opioid use disorder (OUD).

3.1 Understanding Neonatal Opioid Withdrawal Syndrome

Over the past 50 years, there has been a startling rise in the use of prescription and illicit drugs among women and girls during the peak childbearing years, ages 15 to 44. The opioid epidemic has only served to worsen this growing trend among women, which has led to a concurrent rise in the number of births where the child was exposed prenatally to harmful substances, such as alcohol, cocaine, and narcotics [1]. The most salient outcome for the newborn of intrauterine exposure is withdrawal from the illicit or prescribed substance, which typically manifests soon after

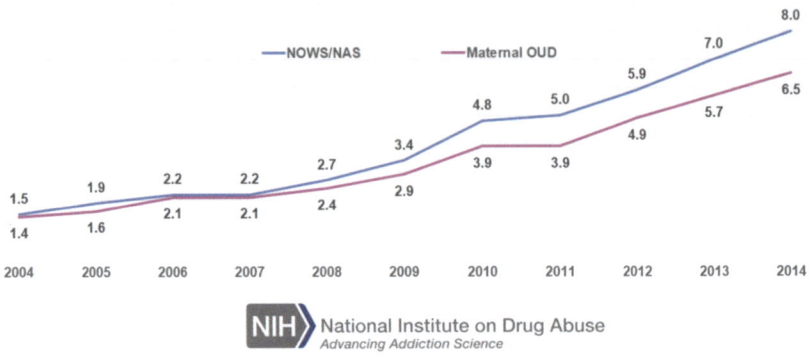

Fig. 3.1 Trends in NOWS and maternal OUD, 2004–2014. This figure shows the parallel rise in maternal opioid use disorder and infants born with neonatal opioid withdrawal syndrome (aka neonatal abstinence syndrome [NAS]). Source National Institute on Drug Abuse. Adapted from Honein et al. Pediatrics. 2019;143(3):e20183801. doi: 10.1542/peds.2018-3801

birth and is marked by a constellation of symptoms, including central nervous system irritability, autonomic nervous system overactivity, and gastrointestinal dysregulation [1, 2].

With the rise in the use of prescription opioids, heroin, and fentanyl among women of reproductive age over the past 30 years, there has been an epidemic in the number of infants born since the turn of the century with NOWS—a subset of neonatal abstinence syndrome (NAS) that refers specifically to withdrawal from opioids [1] (Fig. 3.1). For infants chronically exposed in utero to opioids, the abrupt cessation at birth to the drugs via the placenta results in withdrawal that typically begins within 72 h after birth. Compared with healthy, full-term newborns, infants with NOWS are typically irritable, difficult to console, and have trouble eating and sleeping. They are also more likely to experience a host of medical problems during the birth hospitalization—including intolerance to feedings and respiratory distress.

3.2 The Clinical and Economic Impact of NOWS

For both parents and healthcare providers, the needs of these newborns are high. They typically require extensive monitoring and medical care, including pharmacologic management with morphine, benzodiazepines, and other drugs to ease the withdrawal symptoms—all of which prolong the birth hospitalization.

These associated costs of caring for infants with NOWS are substantial and have risen in tandem with the growing incidence of NOWS births in the United States, increasing nearly ninefold in just over a decade. In 2003, the annual cost of treating NOWS nationally was approximately $61 million (inflation-adjusted US dollars), surging to $316 million by 2012 [3]. By 2016, the latest year for which we have strong data, the associated costs had surpassed half a billion dollars per year ($572.7 million) [4] (Fig. 3.2). A NOWS diagnosis adds

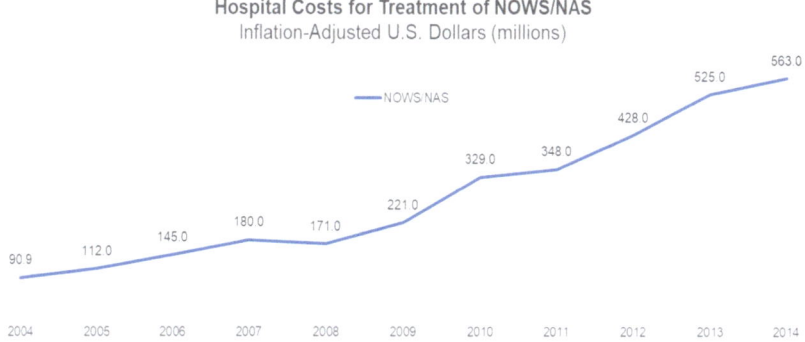

Fig. 3.2 Hospital costs for the treatment of NOWS/NAS, 2004–2014. This figure shows the hospital costs of caring for infants born with neonatal opioid withdrawal syndrome (aka neonatal abstinence syndrome [NAS]) in inflation-adjusted dollars (millions). Source National Institute on Drug Abuse. Adapted from Haight et al. Morbidity and Mortality Weekly Report. 2018

approximately $11,000 to $12,000 to each hospital stay and an additional 15 days, with national data showing median *lengths of stay of 17 days for infants with NOWS, versus less than 2 days for healthy newborns* [3, 5]. In general, the immediate hospital cost of caring for an infant with NOWS is two to five times that of caring for a healthy newborn [3, 6, 7].

Medicaid pays for more than 80% of hospital costs related with NOWS births nationally, placing a substantial burden on state and federal budgets [4], and some states face disproportionate challenges due to higher rates of maternal opioid use and incidence of NOWS. Beyond direct medical costs, the resources required to manage the health of infants with NOWS during the birth hospitalization have placed considerable strain on US hospitals, healthcare providers, and child welfare services. A 2013 study of Child Protective Services (CPS) workers in Massachusetts found they were dedicating more than 10,000 hours monthly just to caring for infants with NOWS—resulting in labor costs for the state in excess of $4.3 million [8]. These costs have not been met with increased funding.

3.3 Beyond the Hospital: Long-Term Challenges for Infants with NOWS

Unfortunately, research shows that the challenges that infants with NOWS, their parents, and their healthcare providers face in the period immediately after birth continue well after discharge. Multiple studies over the past two decades have shown that infants with NOWS are more likely than other newborns to be readmitted to the hospital within the first few months of life [9, 10]. In an analysis of hospital discharge records for nearly 14 million newborns, I found that infants with NOWS were approximately 1.2 times higher than all other newborns to be readmitted to the hospital within 90 days [10].

These findings were particularly stark when examining specific causes of readmission. Even after adjusting for potential confounding factors, such as low birth weight, gestational age, and type of insurance, infants with NOWS had a 58% higher risk of being readmitted for seizures, nearly double the risk of failure to thrive, and an almost *three times higher risk of traumatic brain injuries*. Most concerning were the findings related to *skull fractures, where infants with NOWS had a 3.7 times higher risk of readmission when compared to other newborns*. These patterns of injury raise important questions about the challenges families face in caring for these children at home.

Unfortunately, they were also more likely to be readmitted with a diagnosis of *confirmed* maltreatment (i.e., a diagnosis confirming either abuse, neglect, or both) as opposed to a diagnosis where maltreatment was only suspected. And while other researchers have found that infants with NOWS are at elevated risk of abuse, including physical abuse [11], I found that infants with NOWS were 14 times more likely than other newborns to be readmitted to the hospital within the first 3 months of life for confirmed neglect [10]. The results when it came to physical abuse were not as clear cut or as stark. Prior to controlling for clinical and socioeconomic variables, I found that the risk of a hospital readmission for physical abuse was nearly four times that of other newborns, but once I controlled for these other factors, the results for physical abuse were no longer statistically significant. These findings highlight a critical distinction in the types of child maltreatment risk that may affect families impacted by maternal opioid use. The dramatically elevated risk for neglect, rather than physical abuse, suggests that parents may be struggling with providing adequate care rather than exhibiting intentionally harmful behavior. *This distinction is important for developing appropriate interventions that focus on parental support and education rather than punitive approaches.*

It should be noted, however, that diagnosing physical abuse is particularly challenging. Even so, my research, and that of others, points to a clear risk of neglect in this population and speaks to the stress that mothers and families are under in trying to manage a substance use disorder while also caring for a vulnerable newborn—the care of which may be made more challenging because the infant may still be withdrawing from opioids once home from the hospital. The maltreatment findings are likely a reflection, too, of the difficulties healthcare providers, hospitals, and CPS have in trying to help families transition from home to hospital.

For all families, regardless of whether they are impacted by opioids or not, learning to care for their newborn begins while the child is still hospitalized. Yet, the current standard of care received by most families affected by maternal opioid use leaves them ill-prepared to care for their newborns once they go home. According to Dr. Matthew Grossman, a pediatrician at Yale University and an expert in the care of infants with NOWS, because of the complexity involved in caring for these infants and managing their opioid withdrawal while in the hospital, many of their mothers do not receive the same newborn teaching (e.g., safe sleep, car safety) from healthcare providers that other mothers are given. Even more troubling, mothers who give birth to infants with NOWS are often separated from their newborns during the child's hospital stay.

3.4 Evolving Standards of Care: From Finnegan to Family-Centered Approaches

For nearly 50 years, the standard of care for infants exposed in utero to opioids has been the Finnegan approach. First developed by Dr. Loretta Finnegan in 1975 and later modified by Dr. Lauren Jansson and other practitioners over the years, the Finnegan approach standardizes the management of the care of infants with NOWS by quantifying the withdrawal symptoms [12]. The Finnegan Neonatal Abstinence Scoring Tool (FNAST) is a complex scoring system that prioritizes pharmacologic treatment of the withdrawal symptoms. In all, the full version consists of 21 items, some of which contain subcategories with multiple items that are to be evaluated every 2 to 4 h. For example, the tool assesses whether the infant is experiencing tremors, sweating, or crying excessively. The answers to these questions and the other assessments result in a total score that is then used to determine the type and amount of medications the infant should receive.

Given the complexity involved in regularly monitoring the infant for symptoms and going through the lengthy checklist, it is standard to admit these infants to the neonatal intensive care unit (NICU), which presents physical and psychological challenges for mothers and families during a critical bonding time. Mothers are separated from their newborns, often discouraged from breastfeeding, and, to some extent, even discouraged from holding their infants.

Proponents of the Finnegan approach believe it enables healthcare professionals to quickly assess the infant, identify withdrawal symptoms, and initiate the appropriate medication regimen—the mainstay of which is oral opioids, which serve to replace the opioids the newborn was exposed to in utero, thereby easing the withdrawal symptoms. Infants with a score of eight or higher would then be started on a pharmaceutical regimen that typically involves oral morphine or methadone as first-line therapy that is supplemented as necessary with phenobarbital or clonidine [12, 13].

Others see downsides to the Finnegan approach, and some feel that it leads to the *overmedication of infants and family separation during critical bonding periods.* The level of care mandated by the Finnegan approach is intensive and necessitates that the infant be admitted to the NICU because the care is difficult to institute. This approach is also lengthy and expensive. Whereas healthy newborns are typically discharged within 1 to 2 days, the average length of stay for an infant with NOWS receiving care under the Finnegan approach is 17 days [14].

This level of care is resource-intensive for hospitals and providers. It is also difficult on families. Prior to 2013, infants exposed in utero to opioids were "roomed-in" on a mother-infant unit. Those infants who needed to be observed frequently or who needed medication to soothe their withdrawal symptoms were transferred to the NICU. Once stabilized, infants were typically transferred back to a pediatric floor, enabling families to once again room-in with their child and resume parental care of the infant [14]. What's important to note is that this trajectory of care is based on what worked best for the providers not for the families, who are burdened by having to follow their infants through multiple locations and to hand over the child to teams of providers on a different unit. In a study conducted at Dartmouth University in 2013, families were interviewed about the standard of care with infants with NOWS. Parents reported discontent with the treatment: their infants were awakened from sleep, removed from their arms in order to be assessed by the Finnegan tool, and scored negatively for normal newborn behavior such as crying when hungry [14].

The Finnegan approach has been adopted worldwide and is now the most widely used method for assessing and managing withdrawal symptoms for infants exposed to opioids in utero. But in recent years, because of concerns about the impact of the approach on newborns and their families, new models of care have emerged.

3.5 The Eat, Sleep, Console Approach: A Paradigm Shift

Perhaps the most promising of these new models is one that places the family—mothers in particular—at the center of the child's care. The Eat, Sleep, Console approach was developed in 2014 as part of a larger quality improvement initiative within the Department of Pediatrics at Yale-New Haven Children's Hospital [15]. Led by Dr. Matthew Grossman and a small group of frontline clinicians, this endeavor would fundamentally change how newborns and families affected by maternal opioid use are cared for in the United States.

Dr. Grossman and his team had cared for hundreds of infants with NOWS over the years and saw firsthand the problems posed by the Finnegan approach. The frequency of the FNAST assessments meant that the baby had to be regularly disturbed and unswaddled to elicit signs of withdrawal, and while the scoring tool helped clinicians monitor and manage the symptoms of withdrawal, parents were unhappy. They desired more education. They wanted to know what was happening to their child and sought more direct involvement in their infants' care.

Additionally, because the child was placed in the NICU and the parents were under scrutiny by child welfare agencies, according to Dr. Grossman, they missed out on the basic newborn education that other parents received. Mothers were not allowed to breastfeed due to concerns over drugs passing to the infant through the breast milk. This was true even for those mothers who were considered clinically okay to breastfeed because they were receiving treatment for their opioid use disorder [16].

Dr. Grossman observed that while overall some infants did well on the medications given to ease the withdrawal symptoms, their health began to decline when their mothers were discharged. Grossman asked himself whether the child needed more medication or "more mom."

From the outset, Dr. Grossman and his team set out to develop an approach to NOWS care that moved away from pharmacologic management and returned to a system that revolved around eating, sleeping, and consoling the infant. Parental involvement was not only encouraged but also considered essential. Mothers were encouraged to room-in with their newborns and, for those mothers who were considered stable on methadone or buprenorphine (and not concurrently taking illicit drugs), to soothe them through breastfeeding (or bottle-feeding if breastfeeding was contraindicated). Reflective of the simplicity of the model and the return to the basic principles, the initiative was simply called Eat, Sleep, Console (or ESC). Unlike with the FNAST, only three criteria are assessed with ESC. Is the newborn able to:

1. Breastfeed well (or consume at least 1 ounce of formula)
2. Sleep undisturbed for at least 1 h
3. If irritable, be consoled within 10 min

"Rooming-in" is the core concept of the ESC paradigm [14, 15]. Unless the newborn is critically ill, the goal is to care for all infants with NOWS outside of the NICU. Mothers are encouraged to stay in the same room with their newborns for the child's full hospital stay, and all assessments and treatments are to be carried out in these mother-infant rooms [14, 17], where loud noises and bright lights are kept to a minimum. Gentle handling of the infant is encouraged as is skin-to-skin contact between the mother and newborn.

Under the ESC model, infants are still treated with medications but only after these other measures have been tried first. ESC is a function-based approach that is family-centered. In fact, family empowerment is at the center of this approach, as is education.

In the decade since ESC was developed, it has been adopted worldwide and is becoming the standard of care in many institutions. Although many still rely on the Finnegan or a modified version, hospitals have increasingly adopted the ESC approach, which is not only simpler and more pragmatic, but also more cost-effective. In a study published in 2016, Dartmouth University researchers found that a protocol of rooming-in, on-demand feedings, and skin-to-skin contact for mother and child, as well as family education, resulted in a shorter hospital length of stay for the child [14]. Hospital costs were also lower—in part due to the use of fewer medications and NICU beds.

These results have been corroborated with more recent studies, including a 2023 study funded by the National Institutes of Health (NIH) as part of its ACT NOW (Advancing Clinical Trials for Neonatal Opioid Withdrawal) initiative, which seeks to improve the care of infants exposed to opioids through evidence-based interventions [17]. Specifically, Young et al., in a study directly comparing the Finnegan approach to Eat, Sleep, Console, found that the latter reduced the need for medications and the time until infants were medically ready for discharge—all without compromising the health and safety of the child.

As with Eat, Sleep, Console, the initiatives at Dartmouth and other institutions across the country are simple, pragmatic solutions that revolve around family empowerment, involvement, and education—all of which are critically important. As part of the Dartmouth study, for example—which aimed to improve family-centered care of newborns affected by opioids—in addition to the rooming-in intervention, a program was developed whereby opioid-dependent pregnant women receiving treatment at Dartmouth Hitchcock's perinatal addiction program were given prenatal education to prepare them and their families for the upcoming hospital stay related to their newborns. They were told in advance of what was considered an ideal environment for the child (e.g., low-stimulation), expected length of stay, and what was expected of a consistent family caregiver [14]. At the same time, staff received education on how to skillfully communicate and work with families struggling with opioid addiction.

3.6 Research Gaps and Future Directions

But these initiatives address only a narrow aspect of the crisis: the medical management of infants with NOWS/NAS in the immediate postpartum period. The health and well-being of infants and their families once they are discharged from the hospital have received much less attention. Unlike with the hospital care, there has been no fundamental overhaul of the system to support families in the transition home and in supporting families as they learn to care for a vulnerable (and often challenging) infant in the context of also managing a substance use disorder. Most of the work in this area to date has focused on the complications that infants with NOWS experience while under the care of trained hospital staff.

At present, there are several clinical studies underway at the NIH as part of the ACT NOW coalition [18]. Most of these studies are focused on better understanding Eat, Sleep, Console and the pharmacologic management of infants with NOWS. There is one longitudinal study underway that follows infants for the first 2 years of life, but the aim of this study is to determine to what extent NOWS is associated with adverse neurological and developmental outcomes. Specifically, how do infants exposed to opioids during pregnancy compared to infants who were unexposed in terms of changes to brain structure and connectivity and how do these changes influence medical, behavioral, and developmental trajectories during early childhood? [18] Interestingly, this longitudinal study (Outcomes of Babies with Opioid Exposure or OBOE trial) is also researching the extent to which maternal mental health, the home environment, and parenting have the potential to modify (for better or worse) long-term neurobiological and developmental outcomes [18].

These initiatives are essential and provide valuable insights into how we can improve inpatient care and long-term neurobiological and developmental outcomes for infants with NOWS. Yet, there remains a critical need to understand what happens to these infants and how we can help them once they are home from the hospital.

Likewise, we need to widen our area of concern to the mother and family as a unit. We know that all new mothers are at risk of postpartum depression. Approximately 80% of women will experience mild mood changes in the form of "baby blues" within the first few weeks after giving birth [19]. For approximately one in ten women in the United States, these mood changes will be in the form of postpartum depression, a serious and often debilitating illness [20]. As unthinkable as it is, suicide is a leading cause of maternal mortality in the first postpartum year [21].

3.6 Research Gaps and Future Directions

What happens to mothers when you add a substance use disorder to these mental health challenges? Research has shown that postpartum mothers with an opioid use disorder (OUD) have significantly higher rates of morbidity and mortality compared to the general population. A 2023 study of women receiving public insurance (e.g., Medicaid) showed that fatal opioid overdose rates among postpartum women with OUD are approximately 118 per 100,000 US deliveries [22]. The risk of suicide for these women is estimated at 26 per 100,000 deliveries. Compare these numbers to the risk of death in the general postpartum population: 5.4 per 100,000 deliveries.

For the population as a whole, it is important to note that the majority of deaths among pregnant and postpartum women occur outside of any healthcare setting [23]. This is in contrast to deaths among obstetric decedents in the general population, who primarily die in the hospital. Yet, the majority of pregnant women and postpartum overdose victims die at home or in another nonmedical setting [23].

Infants, in turn, are also at risk due to the stressors experienced by their mothers following hospital discharge. When we look at the risks to children once they are discharged home, we know from prior research that all infants, regardless of whether they are born healthy or exposed in utero to substances, are at risk of maltreatment [24, 25]. (Maltreatment is a broad term that encompasses physical, sexual, and/or emotional abuse as well as neglect.)

Medically, infants with NOWS continue to suffer from many of the problems that affect them during the birth hospitalization and remain irritable and difficult to console after hospital discharge. This intersection between a parent's stress and the child's vulnerability increases the risk of maltreatment for infants with NOWS [10].

In 2024, I completed a study of nationally representative hospital discharge records on nearly 14 million newborns, nearly 90,000 of whom were infants born with NOWS [10]. I found that infants with NOWS had a 3-month hospital readmission rate approximately 1.2 times higher than all other newborns. Even after adjusting for potential confounders, including gestational age at birth, low birth weight, singleton vs. multiple gestation (e.g., twins or triplets), insurance, and year of birth hospitalization, these differences in all-cause readmission rates held true. The data were more concerning regarding the cause of readmission. Infants with NOWS were substantially more likely than other newborns to be readmitted for failure to thrive (a condition where the infant is not growing or gaining weight), seizures, and serious injuries—including for head injuries such as skull fractures and traumatic brain injury [10].

These findings were consistent with other regional and hospital-based studies, which showed that infants with NOWS (or NAS, depending upon the year of the study) had a higher readmission risk than other newborns. Depending upon the study, the reported risk is thought to be 1.5 to 2.5 times higher for infants with NOWS. When it comes to trying to tease out the risk of abuse versus neglect in this population, the results are less clear.

The vulnerability of infants with NOWS extends beyond the early months of life. In a study using child death review data, examining the circumstances surrounding the deaths of children from opioids, I found across all age groups (infants to older adolescents) that 25% had a history of maltreatment [10]. For families struggling with substance use disorders, the challenges of caring for children—especially those with complex medical needs like infants with NOWS—can be overwhelming without adequate support. The pattern of neglect observed in the hospital readmissions data aligns with findings from child fatality review data, where caregiver substance use was a common factor in fatal poisonings of young children. These findings highlight the urgent need for long-term, integrated support for families affected by opioid use disorders, not just during the neonatal period but throughout childhood.

In light of my findings on the circumstances behind fatal pediatric opioid poisonings, it is clear that the vulnerabilities of children extend far beyond any single developmental stage. The patterns of substance use and maltreatment seen across age groups—from infants to teenagers—indicate that our approach to protecting children must evolve beyond isolated interventions. What is needed is a fundamental shift that recognizes opioid exposure as a family-level risk requiring family-centered solutions. As we move toward integrated approaches, we must first address not only the immediate medical needs of these vulnerable children but also the complex interplay of family dynamics, substance use, and child safety that set the conditions for these tragedies.

3.7 Toward Integrated Care Models: Supporting the Mother-Infant Dyad

While the Eat, Sleep, Console approach has transformed inpatient care for families affected by maternal opioid use, significant gaps remain in supporting these vulnerable families once they leave the hospital. For those who do receive care, the treatment is often siloed. Adult substance use treatment rarely considers children in the family, and pediatric care often overlooks parental substance use disorders. This fragmented approach leaves families without the integrated support they need during the critical transition from hospital to home.

Before the child and parents leave the hospital, a checklist should be completed by the healthcare provider that addresses critical safety information and other necessary steps that must be taken to ensure the safety and well-being of not only the child but also the entire family. In his best-selling book, *The Checklist Manifesto*, Dr. Atul Gawande, a neurosurgeon, argues that a checklist is a simple way to consistently and correctly deliver vital information to people [26]. Checklists have been adopted in all types of fields—including aviation and medicine. Of particular note are the surgical checklists that healthcare providers now universally complete preoperatively. The World Health Organization has stated that the surgical checklist, which has become the standard of care across the globe, is the "biggest clinical invention in 30 years."

Given the complexity and critical importance of ensuring the safety of children exposed in utero to substances, I believe a checklist lends itself particularly well to the discharge planning process for families affected by maternal opioid use. Drawing on my own research and work with mother of infants with NOWS and their healthcare providers, I have developed a template (Fig. 3.3) that can be used as a starting guide and adapted as needed. Specifically, the checklist addresses important relationships; community resources; safety measures, such as lockboxes; emergency

Important Relationships

A. Identify at least 3 key people who will provide regular check-ins and that you can contact in the event that your ability to care for your child is compromised by impending drug or alcohol use (i.e., relapse) or the side effects of OUD treatment (e.g., medications such as methadone and Suboxone® may cause drowsiness or mood changes). Ideally, the list should include:
    a. Family member or friend
    b. Neighbor
    c. Trusted healthcare professional
 B. Similarly, create a list of people not allowed in the home when your child is present.
    a. Also, plan for what to do if one of these individuals turns up unexpectedly.

Community Resources

C. Keep a list of important phone numbers on your refrigerator for people/services to call for support. Potential services to include:
    a. Child's pediatrician
    b. Local emergency department
    c. Parenting support groups
    d. 12-step groups or AA (Alcoholics Anonymous) sponsors
    e. Housing or food assistance programs

Safety Measures

D. Proactively prepare your home by:
    a. Storing all opioids in a medication lockbox
    b. Placing doses of Narcan in accessible locations around the home

Emergency Preparations

E. Pack a diaper bag with the essentials you will need in the event that it becomes necessary for you to either leave home with the child or for someone to come and get the child. At a minimum, you should include the following items:
    a. Food
    b. Diapers
    c. Clothes
    d. Toys

Stress and Mood Regulation
F. Make a list of the triggers (e.g., infant crying) that have in the past upset you or caused you to lose your temper.   a. For each trigger, list an action you will take to regain your composure.
Motivation to Stay Sober
G. Make a list of why you should stay sober for yourself and for your child.   a. Similarly, list the potential consequences if you do not stay sober.
Additional Items
H. What other measures can you think of in advance that you can take to keep your infant safe?

Fig. 3.3 Template safety plan. This template is intended to serve as a starting point for helping families affected by maternal OUD with the discharge planning process of mothers. The template addresses several core components (relationships, resources, safety and emergency preparedness, stress, emotional regulation, and motivation to stay sober). The checklist can be tailored to fit a family's particular needs

preparedness, including naloxone access; stress and mood regulation; and motivations to stay sober. And, consistent with the principles Dr. Gawande outlines in his book, the safety plan is simple, concise, and practical. As such, it lends itself to the complex, and often chaotic, environment that surrounds families affected by maternal opioid use.

Caring for a substance-exposed infant is not only medically intensive, requiring extensive resources and personnel, but also the hospital discharge planning is stressful, particularly if CPS (or the Department of Children and Families [DCF], as it is called in some states) is involved. Because of what is often a chaotic environment, families typically miss out on newborn teaching revolving around safe sleeping, use of car seats, etc., leaving them ill-prepared to care for their newborns after hospital discharge.

More than this, though, we are sending highly vulnerable newborns home with parents who are themselves vulnerable and at high risk for substance use or relapse, if they are abstaining. For parents in even the best of circumstances, going home with a newborn is stressful. While this dual vulnerability creates significant risks, existing policy frameworks provide an opportunity for intervention. Plans of Safe Care are federally mandated discharge plans required for infants exposed to substances in utero, designed to ensure both the safety and well-being of the infant and appropriate treatment for the affected family members [27, 28]. Given this existing framework, embedding a checklist into Plans of Safe Care is a logical step forward. In particular, a standardized checklist that is completed prior to discharge would ensure that critical issues are addressed and real objective measures are put in place before the child goes home. Moreover, to avoid stigmatizing mothers and families, the checklist could be applied to all families.

The readmissions identified in my 2024 nationwide readmissions study underscore the dual vulnerability of both the infant with NOWS and the caregiver struggling with an opioid or substance use disorder [10]. The dramatically higher risk of readmission for neglect (14 times higher) compared to other newborns is telling: these families need substantial support to navigate the challenges of caring for a medically complex infant while managing recovery. Rather than viewing these outcomes as evidence of parental failure, we should view them as a reflection of our healthcare system's ability to provide adequate support for the transition from hospital to home. The solutions must be multifaceted, addressing both the medical needs of the infant and the substance use treatment needs of the parents in an integrated, nonstigmatizing manner.

The challenges facing infants with NOWS and their families extend far beyond the initial hospitalization. While significant progress has been made in improving hospital-based care through approaches like Eat, Sleep, Console, there remains a critical gap in supporting these vulnerable families after discharge [15]. A comprehensive approach to care is needed that integrates pediatric care and maternal OUD treatment. By implementing standardized safety checklists and creating models of care that treat the mother-infant dyad, we can begin to address the complex needs of these families. Most importantly, we must move beyond the siloed approach that has characterized treatment to date and embrace collaborative, compassionate models of care that recognize the profound vulnerability of families affected by maternal substance use.

References

1. Patrick SW, Barfield WD, Poindexter BB, Committee on Fetus and Newborn COSUAP. Neonatal opioid withdrawal syndrome. Pediatrics. 2020;146(5). https://doi.org/10.1542/peds.2020-029074.
2. Patrick SW, Schumacher RE, Horbar JD, et al. Improving care for neonatal abstinence syndrome. Pediatrics. 2016;137(5). https://doi.org/10.1542/peds.2015-3835.
3. Corr TE, Hollenbeak CS. The economic burden of neonatal abstinence syndrome in the United States. Addiction. 2017;112(9):1590–9. https://doi.org/10.1111/add.13842.
4. Strahan AE, Guy GP Jr, Bohm M, Frey M, Ko JY. Neonatal abstinence syndrome incidence and health care costs in the United States, 2016. JAMA Pediatr. 2020;174(2):200–2. https://doi.org/10.1001/jamapediatrics.2019.4791.
5. Ko JY, Wolicki S, Barfield WD, et al. CDC grand rounds: public health strategies to prevent neonatal abstinence syndrome. MMWR Morb Mortal Wkly Rep. 2017;66(9):242–5. https://doi.org/10.15585/mmwr.mm6609a2.
6. Winkelman TNA, Villapiano N, Kozhimannil KB, Davis MM, Patrick SW. Incidence and costs of neonatal abstinence syndrome among infants with medicaid: 2004–2014. Pediatrics. 2018;141(4). https://doi.org/10.1542/peds.2017-3520.
7. Jenkins C, Hudnall M, Hanson C, Lewis D, Parton JM. Cost of care for newborns with neonatal abstinence syndrome in a state medicaid program. JAMA Netw Open. 2024;7(2):e240295. https://doi.org/10.1001/jamanetworkopen.2024.0295.
8. Franca UL, Mustafa S, McManus ML. The growing burden of neonatal opiate exposure on children and family services in Massachusetts. Child Maltreat. 2016;21(1):80–4. https://doi.org/10.1177/1077559515615437.
9. Patrick SW, Burke JF, Biel TJ, Auger KA, Goyal NK, Cooper WO. Risk of hospital readmission among infants with neonatal abstinence syndrome. Hosp Pediatr. 2015;5(10):513–9. https://doi.org/10.1542/hpeds.2015-0024.
10. Gaither JR, Drago MJ, Grossman MR, et al. Hospital readmissions among infants with neonatal opioid withdrawal syndrome. JAMA Netw Open. 2024;7(9):e2435074. https://doi.org/10.1001/jamanetworkopen.2024.35074.
11. Puls HT, Anderst JD, Bettenhausen JL, et al. Newborn risk factors for subsequent physical abuse hospitalizations. Pediatrics. 2019;143(2). https://doi.org/10.1542/peds.2018-2108.
12. Finnegan LP, Connaughton JF Jr, Kron RE, Emich JP. Neonatal abstinence syndrome: assessment and management. Addict Dis. 1975;2(1–2):141–58.
13. Finnegan L. Management of maternal and neonatal substance abuse problems. NIDA Res Monogr. 1988;90:177–82.
14. Holmes AV, Atwood EC, Whalen B, et al. Rooming-in to treat neonatal abstinence syndrome: improved family-centered care at lower cost. Pediatrics. 2016;137(6). https://doi.org/10.1542/peds.2015-2929.
15. Grossman MR, Berkwitt AK, Osborn RR, et al. An initiative to improve the quality of care of infants with neonatal abstinence syndrome. Pediatrics. 2017;139(6). https://doi.org/10.1542/peds.2016-3360.
16. Meek JY, Noble L. Section on B. Policy statement: breastfeeding and the use of human milk. Pediatrics. 2022;150(1). https://doi.org/10.1542/peds.2022-057988.
17. Young LW, Ounpraseuth ST, Merhar SL, et al. Eat, sleep, console approach or usual care for neonatal opioid withdrawal. N Engl J Med. 2023;388(25):2326–37. https://doi.org/10.1056/NEJMoa2214470.
18. National Institutes of Health. Advancing Clinical Trials in Neonatal Opioid Withdrawal (ACT NOW). https://heal.nih.gov/research/infants-and-children/act-now. Accessed 4 June 2024.

19. Policy Center for Maternal Mental Health. Maternal Mental Health Disorders. https://policycentermmh.org/mmh-disorders/. Accessed 2 Jan 2025.
20. Khadka N, Fassett MJ, Oyelese Y, et al. Trends in postpartum depression by race, ethnicity, and prepregnancy body mass index. JAMA Netw Open. 2024;7(11):e2446486. https://doi.org/10.1001/jamanetworkopen.2024.46486.
21. Chin K, Wendt A, Bennett IM, Bhat A. Suicide and maternal mortality. Curr Psychiatry Rep. 2022;24(4):239–75. https://doi.org/10.1007/s11920-022-01334-3.
22. Suarez EA, Huybrechts KF, Straub L, et al. Postpartum opioid-related mortality in patients with public insurance. Obstetr Gynecol. 2023;141(4):657–65. https://doi.org/10.1097/AOG.0000000000005115.
23. Han B, Compton WM, Einstein EB, Elder E, Volkow ND. Pregnancy and postpartum drug overdose deaths in the US before and during the COVID-19 pandemic. JAMA Psychiatry. 2024;81(3):270–83. https://doi.org/10.1001/jamapsychiatry.2023.4523.
24. Leventhal JM, Gaither JR. Incidence of serious injuries due to physical abuse in the United States: 1997 to 2009. Pediatrics. 2012;130(5):e847–52. https://doi.org/10.1542/peds.2012-0922.
25. Leventhal JM, Martin KD, Gaither JR. Using US data to estimate the incidence of serious physical abuse in children. Pediatrics. 2012;129(3):458–64. https://doi.org/10.1542/peds.2011-1277.
26. Gawande A. The checklist manifesto: how to get things right. Metropolitan Books; 2010.
27. Bruns LA, Gilmartin ABH, Hannan KE, Hwang SS, Weikel BW. Plans of safe care in substance-exposed infants: components, complexities, and collaboration. Neoreviews. 2025;26(4):e264–73. https://doi.org/10.1542/neo.26-4-005.
28. Deutsch SA, Donahue J, Parker T, Hossain J, Loiselle C, De Jong AR. Impact of plans of safe care on prenatally substance exposed infants. J Pediatr. 2022;241:54–61 e7. https://doi.org/10.1016/j.jpeds.2021.10.032.

The Hidden Crisis: How the Opioid Epidemic Has Endangered America's Children

4

Through an analysis of national hospitalization data, mortality records, and a detailed case review, this chapter examines the profound impact that the opioid crisis has had on children in the United States, a population that is often overlooked in the national discourse. Comprehensive data spanning more than 25 years reveals that more than 15,000 children have died from opioid poisonings in the United States and suggest that another 70,000 have been hospitalized for serious nonfatal exposures. My research documents how the pediatric opioid crisis has evolved from primarily prescription opioid poisonings to today's fentanyl-driven epidemic, which now accounts for 95% of opioid deaths in children. Through a review of nearly 1700 child fatality reports, I highlight recurring patterns across different age groups and family, home, and community factors that place children at risk, including how parental substance use and mental health disorders increase vulnerability. A case study of a 10-month-old who died from fentanyl intoxication despite multiple opportunities for intervention illustrates how system failures and critical gaps in coordination between healthcare providers and child welfare agencies contribute to these preventable tragedies. For families and communities, these findings underscore the extent to which children are at risk from opioids and how practical safety measures can mitigate the risks that opioids pose to children; for healthcare providers, public health officials, and child welfare advocates, they highlight the need for standardized screening methods, prevention protocols, and policy changes. Protecting children from opioid exposure requires both clinical vigilance and community-based solutions that recognize children as central to addressing America's ongoing opioid crisis.

4.1 The Overlooked Victims

When America's opioid epidemic is discussed in the medical literature, policy forums, or the news media, the focus overwhelmingly centers on adults. Yet hidden within this larger crisis is a parallel epidemic affecting our most vulnerable:

children of all ages. Beyond the well-documented impacts on neonates exposed in utero, the broader pediatric opioid crisis remains largely unrecognized. In the span of 25 years, more than 15,000 children have died from opioid poisonings in the United States, and an estimated 70,000 have been hospitalized for serious but nonfatal ingestions.

These morbidity and mortality findings reflect the evolving nature of the opioid crisis: what was once a public health problem primarily among young and middle-aged adult men is now an epidemic taking a toll on Americans across the lifespan. In homes, schools, and communities across the United States, children and adolescents are increasingly exposed to prescription and illicit opioids, often with life-threatening consequences: as my colleagues and I reported in the first national studies to examine trends in pediatric morbidity and mortality from opioid poisonings, hospitalizations in children and adolescents have more than doubled in recent years, and the respective *mortality rate has more than tripled.*

Our initial analysis examined national hospital discharge records for children aged 1 to 19 years, focusing primarily on prescription opioid exposures [1]. Notably, in designing this study, we did not anticipate the risk of fentanyl to young children or the possibility of intentional opioid administration by caregivers—gaps in understanding that reflect how dramatically the crisis has evolved in recent years.

The results from this analysis were unexpected. In the span of just 15 years (1997–2012), pediatric hospitalizations for opioid poisonings in children between the ages of 1 and 19 years increased by *nearly 200%* [1]. And while hospitalization rates increased across all four pediatric age groups (1 to 4, 5 to 9, 10 to 14, 15 to 19 years) examined, the largest increases were seen among the youngest and the oldest children. The majority of poisonings were among teens 15 to 19 years of age, who had the highest annual hospitalization rates across all time points, but it was among the youngest children where we saw the largest increase over time—hospitalization rates increased by more than 205% between 1997 and 2012 among toddlers and preschoolers (i.e., children one to four years of age). In comparison, hospitalization rates among older teens increased by 176% (Figs. 4.1 and 4.2).

For children and adolescents overall, we found that there was a slight decrease in hospitalization rates between 2009 and 2012 [1]. This decrease mirrors trends

4.1 The Overlooked Victims

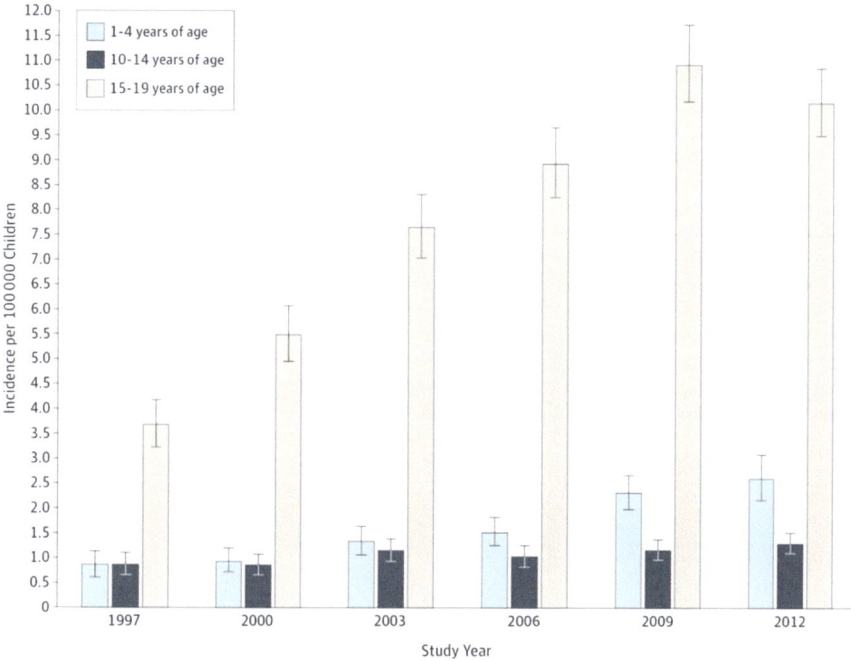

Fig. 4.1 National trends in pediatric hospitalizations for opioid poisonings among children and adolescents, 1997–2012. Weighted national estimates of temporal trends in hospitalizations for prescription opioid poisonings stratified by age category. Error bars indicate 95% CI (*P* for trend, <.001 for all ages). Estimates for 5- to 9-year-olds did not meet the criteria for statistical reliability and thus are not shown. (Source: Gaither et al. [1]. Copyright American Medical Association)

in hospitalizations for opioid overdose seen among adults during this time. As noted by Dart et al., there was a plateau in opioid overdose rates between 2011 and 2013 for the United States as a whole [2]. Both the trends seen in adults and children can be attributed to a slight decrease in the number of opioid prescriptions that were dispensed in the United States during this time (opioid prescribing rates peaked in the United States in 2012 at 81 prescriptions per every 100 people) [3, 4].

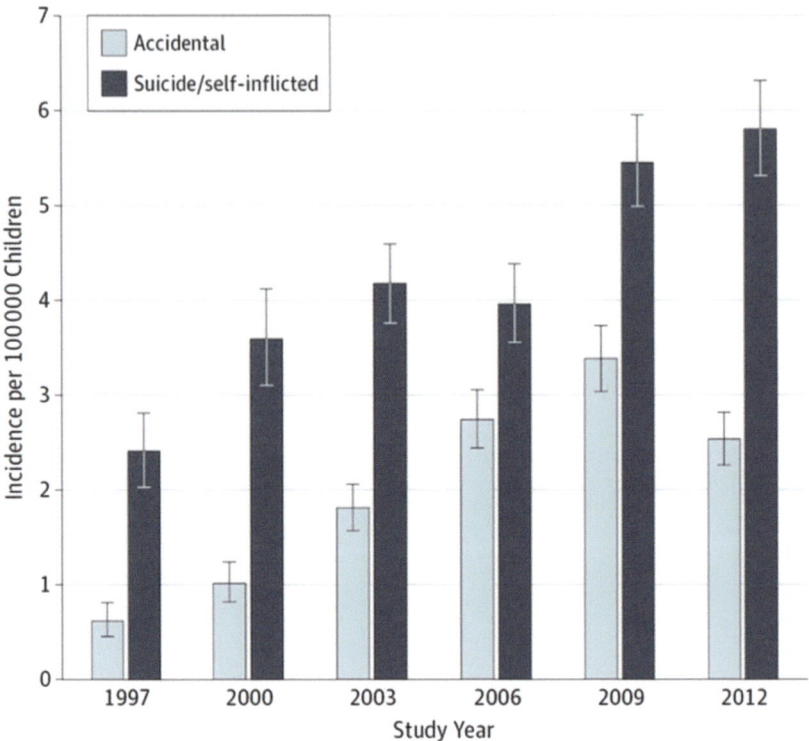

Fig. 4.2 National trends in pediatric hospitalizations for opioid poisonings by intent, 1997–2012. Weighted national estimates of temporal trends in prescription opioid poisonings by intent in the group of 15- to 19-year-olds. Error bars indicate 95% confidence intervals (P for trend, <.001 for poisonings attributed to accidental and suicidal intent). (Source: Gaither et al. [1]. Copyright American Medical Association)

4.2 Changing Patterns in Pediatric Opioid Exposures

When examined by age group, however, it became clear that this positive change was entirely driven by a decrease in nonfatal prescription drug overdoses among older teens—those 15 to 19 years of age. For younger children, hospitalizations continued to rise through the end of the study period, 2012 [1]. Moreover, for older teens, poisonings attributed to heroin continued to rise (Fig. 4.3), as did poisonings from methadone [1], a long-acting opioid that is prescribed primarily for opioid use disorder but is also prescribed to manage chronic pain in adult patients [5]. Methadone is often diverted for illicit use or nonmedical purposes by both teens and adults [6–8]. In fact, methadone is among the most misused of all prescription medications and is often used for purposes other than it was prescribed, such as for recreational use or to enhance the effects of other substances [5]. We found in our study that pediatric hospitalizations involving methadone increased by an astonishing *950% between 1997 and 2012* [1].

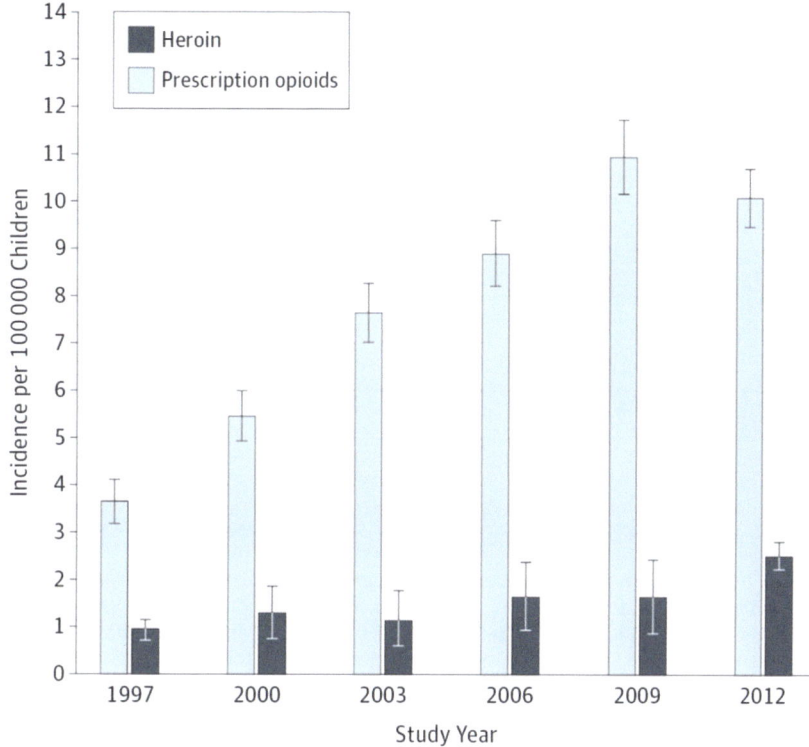

Fig. 4.3 National trends in pediatric hospitalizations for opioid poisonings, heroin versus prescription opioids, 1997–2012. Weighted national estimates of temporal trends in hospitalizations for illicit versus prescription opioid poisonings in the group of 15- to 19-year-olds. Error bars indicate 95% confidence intervals (*P* for trend, <.001 for poisonings attributed to heroin and prescription opioid drug use). (Source: Gaither et al. [1]. Copyright American Medical Association)

Overall, in this study, we found that on average around 2000 children and adolescents were hospitalized a year for nonfatal opioid poisonings, but only about 30 children a year died. But our study focused only on hospitalizations, which was true of most studies at the time. It was only in a subsequent study, which examined in depth deaths from opioids in all settings—medical, residential, and community—that we discovered that the number of children dying from opioid poisonings was actually closer to *500 per year* [9] (Fig. 4.4).

In this first national study to examine pediatric deaths from opioids, my colleagues and I used death certificate data from the Centers for Disease Control and Prevention (CDC) to determine how many children were dying each year from opioid poisonings and how trends had changed since the opioid epidemic began in the late 1990s [9]. At the time, nearly all of what was known concerning opioid deaths came from the adult overdose literature, where it is common practice for researchers to exclude deaths among those younger than 25 years of age.

When researchers do examine deaths among the young, they are typically grouped into two broad categories, such as 0 to 14 and 15 to 24 years. Both practices

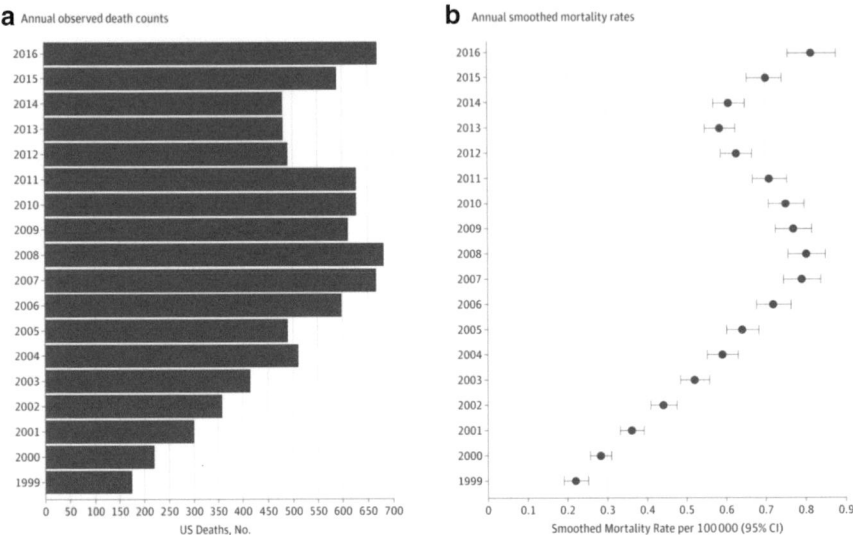

Fig. 4.4 National trends in pediatric deaths from opioids, 1996–2016, annual crude death counts and mortality rates. Number of pediatric mortality rates and number of deaths by year. Number of deaths (**a**) and mortality rates (**b**) for children of ages 0 to 19 years. Error bars indicate 95% confidence intervals. (Source: Gaither et al. [9]. Copyright American Medical Association)

obscure the extent to which the opioid crisis has impacted children and adolescents. For our study, we examined deaths from opioids that had occurred between 1999 and 2016 and included children from infancy up to 20 years of age [9]. And for this study, we examined deaths not only from prescription opioids and heroin but also from fentanyl, a synthetic opioid.

We found that in the span of 18 years nearly 9000 children had died from an opioid poisoning in the United States and that the mortality rate had increased by almost 300% during this time. As with the prior study looking at hospitalizations, we found that while the mortality rate increased in every pediatric age group examined (0 to 4, 5 to 9, 10 to 14, 15 to 19 years), the children most impacted were the youngest and the oldest. Mortality rates increased by 250% among older teens and 225% among the youngest children. For children in the two middle age groups (5 to 9 and 10 to 14 years), mortality rates increased by 100% and 150%, respectively [9] (Fig. 4.5).

One of the most striking findings was where these deaths occurred—over 38% of children died at home, and 62% died outside of any medical facility. This finding is particularly significant given that only 10% died as inpatients, revealing that the majority of pediatric opioid deaths occur in community settings where emergency medical intervention may be delayed or unavailable.

These data also exposed a stark pattern of homicide among the youngest victims—nearly 25% of deaths in children under age 5 were *classified as homicides*, with this percentage rising to 35% among infants. These figures underscore the

4.2 Changing Patterns in Pediatric Opioid Exposures

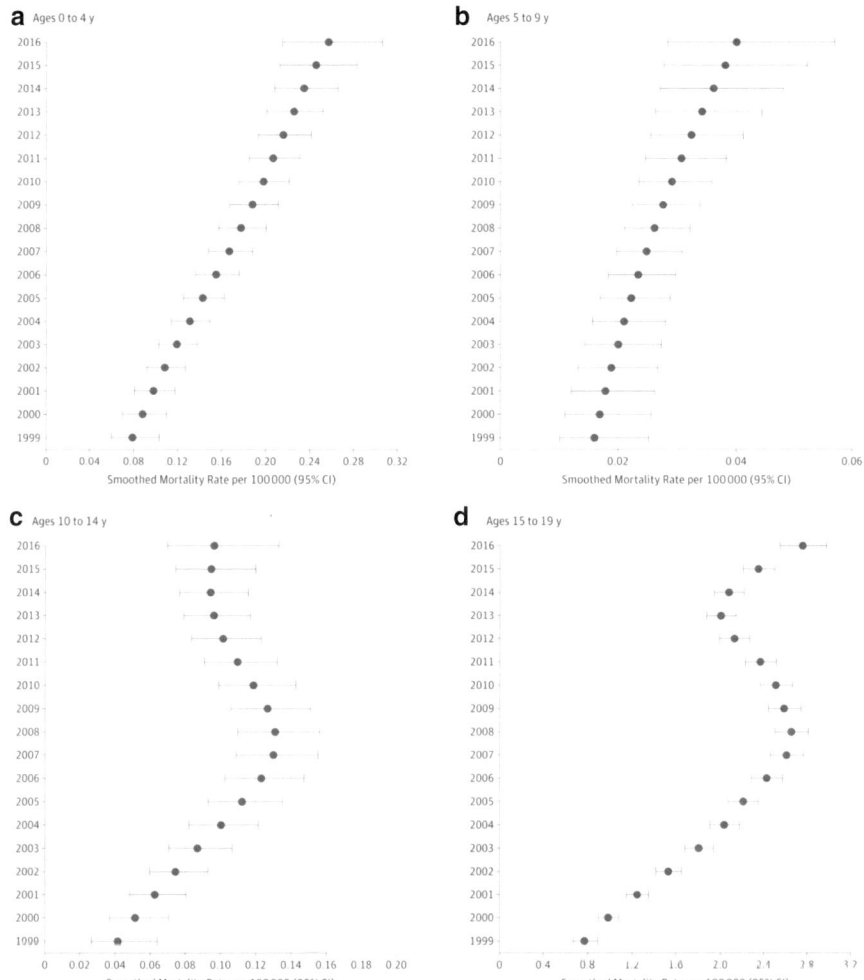

Fig. 4.5 National trends in pediatric deaths from opioids, 1996–2016, annual mortality rates, stratified by age. Age-stratified pediatric mortality rates by year. Deaths in children aged 0 to 4 years (**a**), 5 to 9 years (**b**), 10 to 14 years (**c**), and 15 to 19 years (**d**). Error bars indicate 95% confidence intervals. (Source: Gaither et al. [9]. Copyright American Medical Association)

complex relationship between parental substance use and child safety that remains inadequately addressed by our current child welfare and healthcare systems.

The data also revealed other concerning demographic trends that mirrored trends in the adult population but with unique patterns in children. While white adolescents represented the majority of deaths (80%), Black children experienced the most dramatic percentage increase in mortality—a 391% rise compared to 289% among white children [9]. When examining intent, we found that 81% of all pediatric opioid deaths were classified as unintentional, with only 5% attributed to suicide.

However, among adolescents aged 15 to 19, poisonings involving co-ingestions were alarmingly common—nearly 40% of deaths involved multiple substances, including benzodiazepines (20%), cocaine (12%), and alcohol (7%). These patterns of polysubstance use suggest that prevention strategies must address the complex reality of adolescent experimentation and self-medication rather than focusing solely on opioid access.

In general, we found that whereas the rate of pediatric deaths from opioid poisonings differed from the rate of adult deaths in degree of magnitude, both followed similar trends, which speaks to the systemic nature of the problem and *the influence of adult drug use patterns on children.* For instance, annual pediatric mortality increased steadily through 2008, at which time rates began to decline and essentially plateau from 2012 through 2014. At that point rates began to rise again in response to the emergence of heroin (the second wave of the opioid epidemic) as the opioid of choice for many adults and teens because it was often cheaper and easier to obtain than prescription opioids like OxyContin [2, 10–13].

As noted earlier with the hospitalization study [1], the plateau that occurred between 2012 and 2014 corresponded with the decline in overdose deaths from prescription drugs for the US population as a whole [2]. Again, these trends likely reflect a reining in of the number of opioid prescriptions dispensed during this time as well as the effects of numerous public health measures that were beginning to take effect. Unfortunately, as we all know by now, any public health gains that were achieved from these measures to curtail prescription opioid use were not sustained with the emergence of illegally manufactured fentanyl—the third wave of the opioid epidemic—in the United States [14].

We found for older adolescents that, whereas deaths attributed to prescription opioid poisonings increased 95% over the 18-year study period and deaths from heroin increased by 400%, deaths from synthetic opioids, such as fentanyl, increased by nearly 3000%. Nearly half of these deaths occurred between 2014 and 2016—the final 3 years of the study period [9] (Fig. 4.6).

Fentanyl is a potent synthetic opioid approved by the Food and Drug Administration for relief of severe and/or chronic pain [15]. Fentanyl, like other synthetic opioids (e.g., tramadol), is produced in a laboratory and targets the same receptors in the brain as natural opioids (e.g., morphine and codeine) [16]. Prescription fentanyl comes in liquid, powder, and patch forms.

Yet fentanyl is also manufactured illegally, and it is the illicit form of the drug that is at the root of most overdose deaths. In 2021 alone, it was widely reported in the press that more than 70,000 adults in the United States overdosed on fentanyl [16–18]. A statistic that has received far less attention is that in 2021, there were also nearly 1600 children in the United States who died from fentanyl [19]. In the population-based study of US death certificate data, I analyzed pediatric trends in deaths from fentanyl between 1999 and 2021 using county-level data from the CDC [19]. I focused specifically on deaths among individuals younger than 20 years of age and analyzed the data according to age, demographics, contributing substances, and place and manner of death [19]. In this study, I also examined how the opioid

4.2 Changing Patterns in Pediatric Opioid Exposures

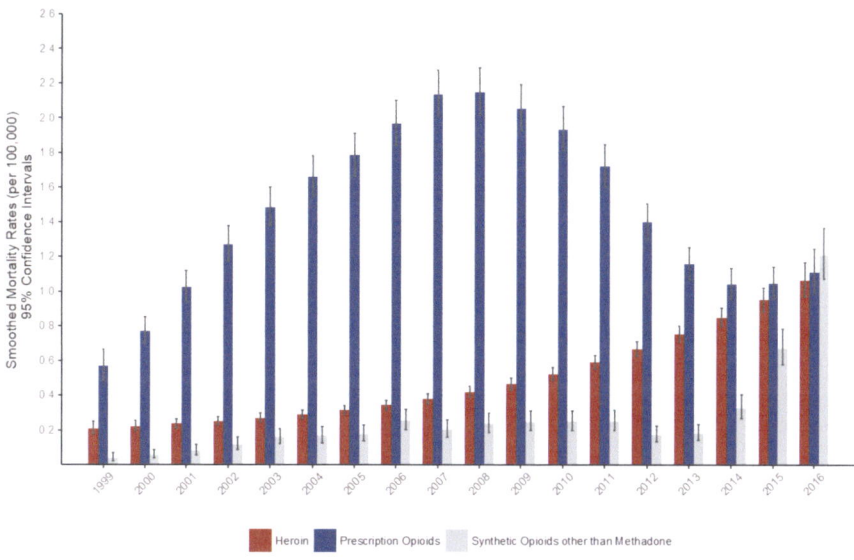

Fig. 4.6 Fatalities for prescription versus illicit opioids, 15–19-year-olds, 1999–2016. Temporal trends in deaths among older teens for prescription compared to heroin and fentanyl. Error bars indicate 95% confidence intervals. (Source: Gaither et al. [9])

epidemic had changed in the years since I began looking at this issue. The results were shocking.

Fentanyl is now responsible for *94% of all pediatric opioid deaths—a stark change from 1999 when only about 5% of pediatric opioid deaths involved fentanyl.* Between 2013 and 2021, fentanyl mortality rates increased more than 30-fold, with a particularly alarming surge beginning in 2018. For children younger than 5, the mortality rate increased by a staggering 590% between 2018 and 2021 alone. In 2021 nationally, fentanyl was responsible for the deaths of 40 infants and 93 children aged 1 to 4 years. Most concerning was the finding that 44% of these deaths occurred in the home; the vast majority (88%) were classified as unintentional (accidental) poisonings [19]. These data underscore that the pediatric opioid crisis is evolving in ways that make it harder to combat with traditional approaches, which primarily focus on prescription medications (Fig. 4.7).

As with adults, it is now clear that fentanyl has become the primary driver of the pediatric opioid crisis. In 1999, the number of deaths from fentanyl among those younger than 10 years of age was fewer than ten (in accordance with the CDC's reporting criteria, the exact number cannot be specified due to privacy concerns for families). But deaths began to increase dramatically in 2013, with a particularly alarming surge that began in 2018. By 2021, all but 100 of the 1657 deaths from opioids that occurred in that year were attributed to fentanyl [19].

Consistent with my earlier research [1], I found again that the majority of deaths were among older adolescents, but astonishingly, in 2021, fentanyl was the cause of death for 133 children younger than age 5. Forty of these children were less than

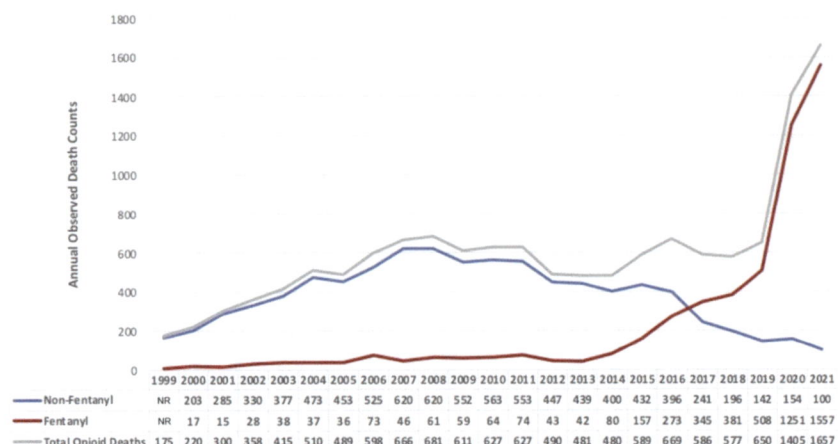

Fig. 4.7 National Trends in Pediatric Deaths from Fentanyl, 1999–2021. Fatal pediatric opioid poisonings stratified by fentanyl versus non-fentanyl, 1999–2021. In accordance with the reporting policies followed by the US Centers for Disease Control and Prevention Wide-Ranging Online Data for Epidemiologic Research, values that would allow for the back calculation of 9 or fewer deaths are not reported (NR). (Source: JAMA Pediatr. 2023;177(7):733–735. doi:10.1001/jamapediatrics.2023.0793. Copyright American Medical Association)

1 year of age. Moreover, whereas between 2018 and 2021, the mortality rate for older teens increased by nearly 300%, it rose by nearly 600% among children younger than 5. That fentanyl now accounts for 94% of fatal pediatric poisonings speaks to the widespread use of fentanyl in society and the lethality of the drug, which is 50 times more potent than heroin and 100 times more potent than morphine [19].

The majority of deaths occurred at home and were attributed to accidents (i.e., unintentional). The largest number of deaths occurred in 2020 and 2021, which suggests that COVID exacerbated what was already a growing public health crisis among children. Not only did substance use among adults and older adolescents increase during COVID, but also with school closure and stay-at-home orders, more children were likely exposed to opioids in the home. With COVID, children considered "at-risk" did not receive the oversight that schools and other agencies normally provide.

A recent study published in the *New England Journal of Medicine* explores nonfatal poisonings in young children from fentanyl, which complements the fatality data I have shown—allowing for a more comprehensive picture of the impact that fentanyl has had on the very young in this country [20]. In an analysis of a decade's worth of data from the National Poison Control Data (2013–2023), Temple and Hendrickson identified 1466 cases of illicit fentanyl exposure among children younger than 6 years of age [20]. Consistent with my work, they found a dramatic rise in annual reports of fentanyl exposure. In 2013, there were five reports; by 2023, there were 539. In the analysis, 84% of the children were 2 years of age or younger, and consistent with my mortality findings, 82% of exposures occurred in the home.

Even in the cases where the exposure was not fatal, the clinical impact was severe: 63% of children had central nervous system depression, and nearly half of children experienced respiratory depression or arrest. Despite medical intervention, for approximately 4% of children, the exposure proved fatal. Together, the fatal and nonfatality findings underscore the need for prevention strategies to protect the youngest among us from fentanyl [20].

4.3 Understanding How Children Die: Circumstances and Classifications

For the pediatric population as a whole, my own research shows that the majority of deaths are from accidental ingestions, and most of these are from prescription medications. Only 5% of pediatric deaths are attributed to suicide and just 2% to homicide [9]. Even among the group with the highest suicide risk—older teens—85% of deaths are deemed accidental (i.e., the intent was not to cause self-harm). Accidental ingestions are also behind a high percentage of deaths in younger children, but among the very youngest, a large proportion are attributed to homicide. Specifically, for children younger than 5, only 38% of deaths are clearly accidental, and one in four deaths are attributed to homicide. For those younger than 1 year of age (i.e., infants), more than one-third of deaths are due to homicide.

It is important to note here that the terms "accidental," "suicide," and "homicide" refer to three of the four official classifications used to categorize the manner of death, with "undetermined representing the fourth classification" [9, 21]. Medical examiners establish manner of death by evaluating the specific circumstances surrounding the death. While the definitions for suicide and undetermined are relatively straightforward, in the context of opioids, accidental poisoning indicates an unintentional or inadvertent exposure. However, the circumstances behind accidental poisonings vary considerably across age groups. For a young child, an accidental poisoning typically involves ingestion of substances encountered in their environment, such as pills found on floors or countertops. In contrast, for teenagers, accidental poisonings commonly occur when recreational drug use results in an unintentional overdose.

The homicide classification also warrants further explanation. Medical examiners categorize a child's death as homicide when the parent or caregiver deliberately acts to harm the child or fails to act appropriately (acts of commission or omission) [22, 23]. Thus, homicide does not necessarily indicate that a parent deliberately harmed their child; it could simply mean that the parent failed to enact basic safeguards to protect the child. To really understand the death of a child, the circumstances that led up to the death must be fully considered.

4.4 Case Study: Marcello's Preventable Death

In the spring of 2024, I received an email from a social worker at the Office of the Child Advocate (OCA) for the State of Connecticut. He was interested in forming a work group to address accidental drug poisonings in children. Between 2020 and 2024, there had been 40 fatal and nonfatal poisonings from fentanyl in the state among children younger than 5. The most prominent case involved the death of a 10-month-old, Marcello, who died on June 28, 2023, from a lethal ingestion of fentanyl and other illicit drugs. Marcello was the 11th child in Connecticut to die from an opioid poisoning since 2020 [22, 24, 25].

Marcello's death was considered a homicide and, pursuant to Connecticut law, the State's Child Fatality Review Panel has a mandate to review the circumstances surrounding the death of any child who had received state services from an agency or department related to child welfare, social services, or juvenile justice. The intent of these reviews is to prevent future tragedies by making recommendations to state agencies regarding needed practice and policy changes.

As intended, the report, which, like all child fatality reports, is a public document available online [22], brought to light the extent to which Marcello's death was preventable and the failures of state agencies to protect Marcello from harm.

Marcello was the second child born to a mother with a long history of opioid misuse and involvement with the criminal justice system. His older sibling, born 3 years earlier, had tested positive for illicit opioids, but the hospital did not fully report the birth to DCF, and no case was opened.

At birth, Marcello tested positive for opioids as well as cocaine and was subsequently diagnosed with neonatal opioid withdrawal syndrome (NOWS) and failure to thrive—a diagnosis that, in conjunction with his NOWS diagnosis, indicated that his early growth and weight gain were compromised. The infant was treated for withdrawal from opioids and received feedings through a nasogastric tube to address the marked weight loss that occurred after birth. Unlike with his sibling, this time the hospital did contact DCF.

The agency created a safety plan to ensure that Marcello and his 3-year-old sibling remained safe as well as to engage their mother in treatment for her substance use disorder. In this context, a safety plan refers to the Child Abuse Prevention and Treatment Act (CAPTA) Plan of Safe Care (POSC) [26]. This federal legislation, which has evolved significantly since its inception in 1974, now requires states to develop safety plans for infants exposed to substances. In Connecticut, like many states, hospitals must submit notifications through a CAPTA portal when an infant is born with prenatal drug exposure, though these reports are often de-identified. The policy framework surrounding these plans—including their effectiveness, implementation challenges, and ongoing policy debates—will be explored in detail in Chap. 5.

Yet, DCF did not conduct adequate assessments and background checks on Marcello's parents. His father was deemed by DCF as the "sober caregiver," even though he, like the mother, had a long history of substance misuse and involvement with the criminal justice system [22]. Most tellingly, while DCF required that the father complete a toxicology screen, he never did so. DCF appropriately referred the mother for home-based substance use treatment, but the in-home treatment provider did not comply with DCF's requirements for drug testing, including fentanyl testing. Records show that the mother received methadone through a treatment facility that required her to travel to the site weekly. Yet, there was no coordination between providers at the facility and DCF regarding safety planning or drug testing.

The few lab tests that were conducted showed that Marcello's mother tested positive multiple times for fentanyl. But after just two negative tests, the in-home treatment provider inaccurately documented that the mother had met the criteria for discharge, even though a minimum of 12 negative tests were actually required for successful discharge per company policy. Citing the mother's successful completion of substance use treatment by the mother, DCF closed its case with the family on June 7, 2023. Marcello was found dead at a relative's home where the mother was staying on June 28, 2023. Toxicology tests ordered by the Office of the Chief Medical Examiner showed that the 10-month-old had ingested a lethal combination of fentanyl, cocaine, and xylazine. A post-mortem investigation revealed evidence of drug use in the bedroom where the mother slept with the children, including drug paraphernalia and Ziplock bags containing fentanyl [24, 25].

The 26-page report by the OCA faults the probation system, DCF, and the substance use providers—both the in-home and methadone providers [25]. In general, there was a lack of communication between agencies and a failure to follow established procedures, particularly related to drug testing and safety planning.

According to federal policy, substance exposure alone is insufficient grounds to substantiate a claim of child abuse or neglect. Given that DCF does not know the identity of the newborn, much is riding on the POSC. These plans are intended to be a family-centered and family-friendly approach to protecting the safety of the child and addressing the needs of families affected by maternal substance use. Considered less punitive, disruptive, and stigmatizing than traditional DCF involvement, POSC are considered compassionate and nonpunitive in that the outlined plans are voluntary; families are not required to follow the recommendations [27].

In Marcello's case, safety planning should have addressed specific protocols for drug testing and supervised visitation. However, the fundamental problem extends beyond this individual case. Despite their widespread adoption, there is little evidence that POSC effectively protect children. As Sarah Font, an associate professor of sociology and public policy at Pennsylvania State University, explains in a recent article published by the American Enterprise Institute, "The term 'plan' implies a set of objectives or steps that will be implemented, but a POSC can be nothing more than a form that documents services the mother or infant already received or were referred to. The voluntary nature of the POSC may mean that the vast majority of parents eligible for a POSC receive no substance use treatment, as studies in New Mexico and Delaware found" [27].

To illustrate Dr. Font's point, below is the entirety of the POSC that was created by DCF for Marcello:

> Mother will not be left alone unsupervised while caring for the newborn child. Mother will continue to actively engage in treatment [with methadone provider]. Mother will utilize father, family, friends, and other natural support to supervise her. DCF will do home visits twice per week.

As noted in the report by the OCA following Marcello's death, the "plan" did not specify how the mother of an infant and a 3-year-old child was to be continuously supervised. She and the baby's father did not live with relatives, and the father was employed outside the home. No family members were specifically identified to provide "natural support." Most importantly, the plan did not address how it would be monitored and the family assessed, including how the parents would be evaluated to ensure that they were not exposing their children to lethal drugs, including fentanyl. Despite the vagueness of the plan and the lack of concrete steps, Marcello was discharged into his mother's care. There was no effective plan to keep Marcello safe, and he died as a result.

The OCA fatality report highlighted critical gaps in safety planning and recommended comprehensive reforms to DCF protocols, including enhanced drug testing requirements, improved information interagency communication, better assessment of caregivers, and more structured monitoring processes. However, as I will discuss further in Chap. 5, these recommendations still fall short of addressing the fundamental challenge: establishing clear protocols for when children should be removed from homes when parents test positive for lethal substances like fentanyl.

4.5 System Failures and Missed Opportunities

Unfortunately, the circumstances surrounding the death of Marcello are consistent with the deaths of hundreds of children across the United States in recent years from opioids in general and fentanyl specifically. In an effort to better understand how and why children die from opioids, I recently completed an analysis of records on children younger than 18 years of age who had died from an opioid poisoning between 2004 and 2020 [28]. This study revealed troubling patterns of family vulnerability and risk factors. Regardless of the age of the child, there were several common themes that echo the circumstances that played a role in the death of Marcello: specifically, system and treatment failures; poor coordination between and among healthcare providers, probation services, and child welfare workers; and family, home, and community risk factors.

More than 65% of the fatalities occurred in the child's own home, and nearly one in four occurred in the home of a relative, friend, or foster parent [28]. The source of the opioid was typically the parents' prescription or illicit drug, a finding that

4.5 System Failures and Missed Opportunities

points to the drugs being kept in unsecured locations. While prescription opioids contributed to 92% of deaths in this study, heroin and illicit fentanyl played an increasingly important role, contributing to 5% and 8% of deaths, respectively. Importantly, 43% of deaths involved another substance, such as antidepressants, benzodiazepines, and/or alcohol. These data are consistent with what national epidemiological data show. But while national data are important for examining trends and giving us a sense of the magnitude of the problem, they are less helpful when it comes to understanding how children die from opioids.

What I learned from this study of nearly 1700 children, which drew from birth and death certificates, medical and autopsy reports, and legal and child welfare records, is the extent to which substance use—whether on the part of the parent or an older teen—and a history of maltreatment were pervasive across age groups. Among 15–17-year-olds, nearly three in four had a history of substance use or abuse. Surprisingly, substance use was prevalent among adolescents in the 10–14-year-old range, where 42% were known to have a positive history. For the youngest children, those 0 to 4 years, nearly half had a parent or caregiver with a history of substance abuse. Many of these younger children had caregivers who were impaired by drugs or alcohol at the time of the child's death, creating situations of extreme vulnerability for the child.

This pattern mirrors what I found in my earlier research of pediatric hospitalizations for opioid poisonings [1]. Whereas teens aged 15 to 19 years consistently had the highest hospitalization rates, the most dramatic percentage increase (205%) occurred among children aged 1 to 4 years. The intent behind these poisonings also revealed troubling patterns—among adolescents of age 15 to 19 years, hospitalizations attributed to suicide or self-inflicted injury increased by 140% over the study period (1997–2012), while accidental poisonings increased by 303%. These findings reveal two simultaneous crises within the pediatric population: increasing environmental exposure among young children and alarming rates of deliberate misuse among adolescents, often intertwined with mental health struggles.

The fatality cases, however, exposed an additional layer of vulnerability. In my analysis of the circumstances behind the nearly 1700 opioid fatalities, the findings regarding maltreatment were alarming. In each age group, at least 25% had a history of maltreatment [28]. Among children younger than age 5, more than one-third of the deaths were classified as homicide, which speaks to the extreme vulnerability of the very young. Approximately 13% of children in this study had previously been placed outside of their homes, and 9% had an open case with CPS at the time of death. More troubling still, 21% of children had a caregiver with a documented history as the perpetrator of maltreatment for either the deceased child or another child in the family.

In all, these findings underscore the need for a comprehensive, multifaceted approach to preventing pediatric deaths from opioids. Interventions that improve how opioids are stored and disposed of should be universal for families who have opioids in the home—whether prescribed or illicit. Universal access to naloxone is also critical, particularly for high-risk families. However, given that nearly half of all deaths included a co-ingestion of another substance (e.g., benzodiazepines), naloxone alone cannot be viewed as an all-encompassing solution as it only reverses the effects of opioids. Even when families are educated about opioid risks or have access to naloxone, the presence of multiple substances complicates both prevention efforts and emergency treatment, highlighting why single-focus initiatives often fail to protect children. My research consistently shows that co-poisonings are pervasive across all age groups, pointing to a critical blind spot in our current approach.

In general, the data highlight the common themes found among pediatric opioid fatalities and the extent to which family and home risk factors affect children at different ages. Prevention strategies must account for these age-specific risks. Particularly surprising was the finding that 42% of children aged 10 to 14 years who died from an opioid poisoning had their own history of substance use—a fact that points to the need for earlier screening and intervention with younger adolescents [28]. Importantly, better coordination is needed between child welfare services and healthcare providers—including those who treat substance use disorders in adults.

4.6 Implications for Policy and Practice

These deaths represent not just statistics, but also families and communities forever changed by tragedy—which are almost always preventable. When we fail to consider children in our response to the opioid epidemic, we overlook critical intervention points that could save lives across generations. By understanding these patterns, we can identify critical opportunities for intervention and develop targeted strategies to protect the most vulnerable.

The data and case studies presented in this chapter reveal a sobering reality: children have become silent casualties in America's opioid epidemic. The evolution of the pediatric opioid crisis mirrors that of adults but with unique vulnerabilities that demand specific attention. From infants experiencing withdrawal at birth to teenagers experimenting with prescription medications, the patterns of exposure vary by age but share common threads of adult substance use, inadequate safeguards, and systemic failures.

As we will see in the next chapter, addressing this pediatric crisis requires a fundamental shift in how we conceptualize and respond to the broader epidemic. The traditional adult-focused approach has failed to protect the young in this country, suggesting that effective solutions must place children at the center of our public health response rather than treating them as secondary considerations. The insights from this research indicate specific intervention points across multiple systems—healthcare, child welfare, substance use treatment, and family support that must be strengthened and better coordinated if we are to prevent future tragedies like the one that led to the death of Marcello.

References

1. Gaither JR, Leventhal JM, Ryan SA, Camenga DR. National trends in hospitalizations for opioid poisonings among children and adolescents, 1997 to 2012. JAMA Pediatr. 2016;170(12):1195–201. https://doi.org/10.1001/jamapediatrics.2016.2154.
2. Dart RC, Surratt HL, Cicero TJ, et al. Trends in opioid analgesic abuse and mortality in the United States. N Engl J Med. 2015;372(3):241–8. https://doi.org/10.1056/NEJMsa1406143.
3. Centers for Disease Control and Prevention. Changes in opioid prescribing practices. https://archive.cdc.gov/www_cdc_gov/drugoverdose/deaths/prescription/practices.html. Accessed 15 Aug 2025.
4. USAFacts. The opioid crisis in data. https://usafacts.org/articles/opioid-addiction-deaths-and-treatment-latest-analysis-data/. Accessed 15 Aug 2025.
5. National Drug Intelligence Center. Methadone fast facts: questions and answers. https://www.justice.gov/archive/ndic/pubs6/6096/index.htm#:~:text=To%20Top-,Is%20abusing%20methadone%20illegal?,severe%20psychological%20or%20physical%20dependence. Accessed 15 Aug 2025.
6. Miech RA, Johnston LD, Patrick ME, O'Malley PM. Monitoring the future: national survey on drug use, 1975–2024: overview and detailed results for secondary school students. https://monitoringthefuture.org/results/annual-reports/. Accessed 15 Aug 2025.
7. National Drug Intelligence Center. Methadone diversion, abuse, and misuse: deaths increasing at alarming rate. https://www.justice.gov/archive/ndic/pubs25/25930/index.htm. Accessed 15 Aug 2025.
8. Jones CM, Baldwin GT, Manocchio T, White JO, Mack KA. Trends in methadone distribution for pain treatment, methadone diversion, and overdose deaths – United States, 2002–2014. MMWR Morb Mortal Wkly Rep. 2016;65(26):667–71. https://doi.org/10.15585/mmwr.mm6526a2.
9. Gaither JR, Shabanova V, Leventhal JM. US national trends in pediatric deaths from prescription and illicit opioids, 1999–2016. JAMA Netw Open. 2018;1(8):e186558. https://doi.org/10.1001/jamanetworkopen.2018.6558.
10. Cicero TJ, Ellis MS. Abuse-deterrent formulations and the prescription opioid abuse epidemic in the United States: lessons learned from OxyContin. JAMA Psychiatry. 2015;72(5):424–30. https://doi.org/10.1001/jamapsychiatry.2014.3043.
11. Compton WM, Jones CM, Baldwin GT. Relationship between nonmedical prescription-opioid use and heroin use. N Engl J Med. 2016;374(2):154–63. https://doi.org/10.1056/NEJMra1508490.
12. Centers for Disease Control and Prevention. Understanding the opioid overdose epidemic. https://www.cdc.gov/overdose-prevention/about/understanding-the-opioid-overdose-epidemic.html. Accessed 15 Aug 2025.
13. Cicero TJ, Ellis MS, Surratt HL, Kurtz SP. The changing face of heroin use in the United States: a retrospective analysis of the past 50 years. JAMA Psychiatry. 2014;71(7):821–6. https://doi.org/10.1001/jamapsychiatry.2014.366.
14. Centers for Disease Control and Prevention. Understanding the epidemic. https://www.cdc.gov/drugoverdose/epidemic/index.html. Accessed 3 Feb 2019.
15. Centers for Disease Control and Prevention. Fentanyl. https://www.cdc.gov/overdose-prevention/about/fentanyl.html. Accessed 15 Aug 2025.
16. Walter K. Fentanyl overdose. JAMA. 2022; https://doi.org/10.1001/jama.2022.22462.
17. Centers for Disease Control and Prevention. Fentanyl. https://www.cdc.gov/opioids/basics/fentanyl.html. Accessed 8 Dec 2022.
18. Centers for Disease Control and Prevention. US overdose deaths in 2021 increased half as much in 2021 – But are still up 15%. https://www.cdc.gov/nchs/pressroom/nchs_press_releases/2022/202205.htm#:~:text=Reported%20and%20predicted%20provisional%20

counts%20of%20drug,the%20numbers%20of%20these%20deaths%20due%20to. Accessed 15 Aug 2025.
19. Gaither JR. National trends in pediatric deaths from fentanyl, 1999–2021. JAMA Pediatr. 2023; https://doi.org/10.1001/jamapediatrics.2023.0793.
20. Temple C, Hendrickson RG. Increasing exposure of young children to illicit fentanyl in the United States. N Engl J Med. 2024;390(10):956–7. https://doi.org/10.1056/NEJMc2313270.
21. National Center for Health Statistics. Vital statistics reporting guidance. A reference guide for completing the death certificate for drug toxicity deaths. https://www.cdc.gov/nchs/data/nvss/vsrg/vsrg02-508.pdf. Accessed 18 Aug 2025.
22. State of Connecticut. Office of Government Accountability. Office of the Child Advocate. Fatality investigations. https://portal.ct.gov/oca/reports-and-investigations/fatality-investigations/oca-fatality-reports. Accessed 1 Sept 2024.
23. New York City Administration for Children's Services. Systemic child fatality review 2022 Annual report. https://www.nyc.gov/assets/acs/pdf/data-analysis/2022/annual-child-fatality-report.pdf. Accessed 18 Aug 2025.
24. State of Connecticut. Office of the Child Advocate. Child fatality investigation executive summary – the Death of Marcello M. from Fentanyl Intoxication – February 2024. https://portal.ct.gov/-/media/OCA/OCA-Recent-Publications/OCAMarcelloExecSummary.pdf. Accessed 18 Aug 2025.
25. State of Connecticut. Office of the Child Advocate. Child fatality findings and recommendations – February 2024. https://portal.ct.gov/-/media/OCA/OCA-Recent-Publications/OCAMarcelloFatalityReviewFinalReport2024.pdf. Accessed 18 Aug 2025.
26. Sieger MHL, Nichols C, Chasnoff IJ. Child Abuse Prevention and Treatment Act, family care plans and infants with prenatal substance exposure: theoretical framework and directions for future research. Infant Child Dev. 2022;31(3) https://doi.org/10.1002/icd.2309.
27. American Enterprise Institute. The US is Failing Substance-Exposed Institute. https://www.aei.org/research-products/report/the-us-is-failing-substance-exposed-infants/. Accessed 28 July 2024.
28. Gaither JR, McCollum S, Bechtel K, Leventhal JM, Mintz S. The circumstances surrounding fatal pediatric opioid poisonings, 2004–2020. Pediatrics. 2024;154(Suppl 3). https://doi.org/10.1542/peds.2024-067043N.

A Systemic Crisis: Failed Responses and Overlooked Solutions

5

America's response to the opioid epidemic over the past three decades has been fragmented and focused primarily on adults in isolation of their families. Little attention has been paid to the risks that children face from opioids, which has resulted in thousands of preventable pediatric fatal and nonfatal poisonings. Drawing on research showing that over 60% of pediatric opioid deaths occur outside medical settings—with nearly 40% in the home—this chapter highlights critical policy failures that have put children at risk. These include the Food and Drug Administration's (FDA) inadequate regulatory response to the dangers opioids pose to children, problematic changes to methadone take-home policies during COVID, and the absence of emergency response training for families. The United States' fragmented healthcare system treats addiction as an individual disease rather than a family issue, creating dangerous blind spots in our national response.

5.1 The Fragmented Response: Individual Solutions for a Family Problem

Despite decades of government interventions, medical advances, and billions in funding, America's opioid epidemic continues to claim lives across generations. While previous chapters documented the toll on children, this chapter addresses a fundamental question: how did we reach the point where children are dying from prescription painkillers, heroin, and fentanyl? [1, 2]. *The answer lies in our fragmented, adult-focused approach to the crisis.*

Across the United States, the same scenarios play out repeatedly. Parents typically receive opioid prescriptions without being warned of the dangers they pose to children or any guidance on safe storage and disposal, and many formulations, such as the fentanyl pain patch and Suboxone sublingual strips, present packaging and disposal challenges that standard child-resistant packages do not address [3–5]. There is also little coordination or communication between those who care for

© The Author(s), under exclusive license to Springer Nature Switzerland AG 2026
J. R. Gaither, *Living with Opioids*, https://doi.org/10.1007/978-3-031-95820-5_5

adults with opioid use disorder and those who are responsible for ensuring the safety and well-being of children.

The fragmented response to the opioid crisis is pervasive. Researchers, healthcare professionals, and public health and government officials have failed to understand that when an adult brings an opioid into the home, everyone in the family is at risk. Public health campaigns target adult users without educating caregivers about protecting their homes, and virtually all of the hundreds of local, state, and federal measures enacted in recent years to contain the epidemic focus on adults. This explains why, after thousands of initiatives and interventions, the United States continues to see rising pediatric exposures to the entire range of opioids, from medications prescribed for legitimate pain to the illicit substances that have flooded communities in recent years.

The roots of this fragmented approach lie in the longstanding failure to recognize the extent to which the pediatric community has been harmed by opioids [1, 2, 6–9]. Prior to my studies on pediatric morbidity and mortality referenced earlier, which were published in 2016 and 2018 [2, 6], respectively, virtually all research on fatal and nonfatal opioid overdoses in the United States focused on adults.

We now know after years of systematically examining the pediatric data that opioid exposures in children directly mirror adult patterns. While pediatric poisoning rates differ from adult overdose rates in degree of magnitude, both follow remarkably similar trends, underscoring the systemic nature of the crisis. Pediatric mortality rates increased steadily from 1999 through 2008 before starting to decline, mirroring broader US trends in opioid prescribing, which peaked in 2010 [10]. Rates began to rise again in response to the emergence of heroin (the second wave of the opioid epidemic) as the opioid of choice for many adults because it was often cheaper and easier to obtain than prescription opioids like OxyContin [2, 11]. These patterns in opioid prescribing are dramatically reflected in older adolescents (15- to 19-year-olds), where any public health gains made in response to the decrease in the availability of prescription opioids have not been sustained with the emergence of heroin around 2011 and illicitly manufactured fentanyl in 2014 [1]. Between 1999 and 2016, prescription opioid fatalities increased by 95%, while heroin overdoses rose by more than 400% and deaths from synthetic opioids (e.g., fentanyl) by nearly 3000% [1].

The public health initiatives tried in the United States to contain the opioid epidemic have often failed because they target isolated aspects of the epidemic rather than the system holistically.

5.2 Failed Policy Initiatives

Consider the efforts that have gone toward changing physician prescribing practices. Physicians are prescribing opioids for pain management less than they were at the beginning of the opioid crisis, but only moderately so [12]. Furthermore, as noted in Chap. 2, as limits have been placed on access to prescription opioids, patients have turned to illicit forms of the drug. Similarly, prescription drug monitoring programs have been implemented to limit the volume of opioids prescribed to patients and to limit the phenomenon of doctor shopping, whereby patients visit multiple doctors to maximize the number of prescriptions they can obtain for the same condition. While these measures did slow the rise in rates of fatal opioid overdoses among adults, they failed to account for the influx of illicit drugs to take the place of prescription pills. Moreover, these efforts fail to address the fundamental issue of how to safely store and dispose of the opioids that are prescribed and those obtained illicitly.

The siloed nature of the US response to the opioid crisis can be seen in the lack of attention to the risks to children during the peak years of the epidemic. My research on pediatric hospitalizations revealed a 950% increase in adolescent hospitalizations for methadone poisonings from 1997 to 2012—likely a direct consequence of the risks that medication-assisted treatment (MAT) posed to children in the household [6]. Moreover, although pediatric hospitalizations for opioid poisonings decreased slightly between 2009 and 2012, heroin poisonings among adolescents continued to rise. This pattern illustrates how interventions focused solely on prescription practices failed to address the progression from prescription opioids to illicit drugs among vulnerable youth.

5.3 Poor Quality of Care: Failure to Follow Prescribing Guidelines

The failure to protect patients from opioids can be seen not only in regulatory failures but in clinical practice itself. In my earliest research on the opioid crisis, I explored the quality of care delivered to US veterans (a group with a high prevalence of pain and substance use disorders) who were prescribed opioid therapy for chronic noncancer pain [13, 14]. This work provides compelling evidence of how, early on in the opioid crisis, healthcare systems failed to implement even basic safety measures for opioid prescribing.

In this study of nearly 21,000 US veterans receiving long-term opioid therapy (3 months or more) between 1998 and 2010, my colleagues and I found alarming gaps in recommended care and actual clinical practice [13]. On average, patients received no more than 40% of care recommended at the time by leading medical societies, including the American Pain Society and the American Academy of Pain Medicine [15]. Even more concerning, this implementation gap persisted despite repeated updates to the guidelines over the decade studied [16].

The findings were particularly concerning regarding high-risk prescribing. Despite clear recommendations against concurrent prescribing of opioids and sedatives due to increased overdose risk, approximately 20% of patients received benzodiazepines along with their opioid medications [13, 17]. Even more troubling was that among patients with an active substance use disorder—approximately 20% of the sample—only half were engaged in substance use treatment [17], directly contradicting recommendations from the clinical practice guidelines [15, 16].

When we examined metrics related to patient monitoring for safety issues and adverse effects, we found that only about half of patients had a primary care visit within 1 month of starting opioid therapy, and urine drug testing—a critical safety measure to assess for opioid misuse—was performed in fewer than 15% of patients [13]. The findings demonstrate that even in a healthcare system with relatively robust oversight and integrated electronic health records, guideline-concordant care remained the exception rather than the rule.

Perhaps most concerning was the persistence of these patterns over time. Despite increasing awareness of opioid risks and multiple updates to the guidelines during the study period, we observed only modest improvements in critical areas of practice, such as decreased coprescribing of benzodiazepines [14], while other high-risk practices, such as prescribing opioids to patients with untreated substance use disorders, actually increased.

Most important, our research found that these lapses in care had real-world consequences [14]. Our analysis of all-cause mortality revealed that patients prescribed benzodiazepines concurrent with opioids had nearly a 40% higher risk of death, while patients with untreated substance use disorders had more than double the mortality risk compared to patients who were receiving treatment for their disorder [14].

These findings highlight how the crisis extends beyond issues of access or regulation to the fundamental question of how healthcare for opioid treatment is delivered. When clinicians fail to follow evidence-based guideline for the safe use of these medications, patients and their families are placed at unnecessary risk. The implementation gap between what we know about safe opioid prescribing and what actually happens in clinical practice is one of the most significant yet overlooked aspects of America's opioid crisis.

5.4 The Heightened Risks of Opioids for Patients with Substance Use Disorders

These gaps in quality of care for patients prescribed opioids for an extended period become more consequential when we consider patients with substance use disorders. In a subsequent study to those outlined above, I expanded on my initial findings to examine how substance use disorders affect mortality risk [17].

In the same population of adult patients, my colleagues and I found that approximately 20% of patients receiving opioids for 30 days or more met the criteria for an active (current) substance use disorder [14, 17]. For these high-risk patients, I found the receipt of mental health services (such as cognitive behavioral therapy) to be particularly protective, reducing mortality risk by nearly 60% compared to a reduction of 35% for those without a disorder. This differential effect demonstrates that mental health support is potentially life-saving for vulnerable patients.

Most concerning was our discovery related to treatment patterns for those with a substance use disorder. We found that only half of patients were engaged in treatment for their disorder—despite clear guidelines recommending against the use of opioids for patients with an untreated disorder. These patients had a mortality risk nearly twice that of those who were receiving appropriate substance use treatment. As noted earlier, in this sample, patients were frequently prescribed benzodiazepines. *Patients with and without active substance use disorders were prescribed opioids at comparable rates.*

These findings underscore the extent to which patients with complex conditions often receive fragmented care. The siloed nature of the current US healthcare system means that pain management, mental health services, and addiction treatment are often delivered in isolation from one another—if they are delivered at all. When providers fail to screen or address substance use disorders in patient receiving opioids, or when they prescribe potentially lethal medication combinations, they place vulnerable patients at significantly higher risk of death.

5.5 Racial Disparities in Opioid Monitoring

In my research, I have also discovered troubling evidence of racial disparities in how clinicians monitor patients who are prescribed opioids. In a study involving 15,000 Black and white patients who were receiving opioid therapy through the VA, my colleagues and I found striking differences in both monitoring practices and how physicians responded when urine drug tests revealed illicit drug use alongside prescribed opioids [18].

While only about 20% of patients received a urine drug test within the first 6 months of treatment with opioids—a period when the risk of overdose is particularly high—*Black patients were nearly twice as likely as white patients to be tested.* This disparity persisted even after controlling for other clinical factors, such as substance use or mental health history.

Among those who received a urine drug test that came back positive, Black patients were disproportionately more likely to have their opioids discontinued when compared to white patients. For instance, among those testing positive for cannabis, *Black patients were more than twice as likely to have their opioids stopped.* The findings were more pronounced when it came to testing positive for cocaine: Black patients were *three times more likely to have their opioids discontinued.*

These findings highlight how clinician bias can manifest in pain management decisions, particularly when clinical guidelines lack clarity. Guidelines recommend monitoring for illicit drug use but provide limited direction on how to respond when tests are positive. The disparities we documented reinforce the need for both universal application of safety monitoring and clearer guidelines for how healthcare providers should respond to evidence of illicit drug use. A more standardized approach—where all patients receive consistent monitoring and follow-up—could help reduce disparities in care.

These failures in clinical practice represent only part of the problem, however. As we will see next, regulatory failures have further compounded opioid risks by failing to provide adequate safeguards to protect vulnerable patients.

5.6 Regulatory Failures

The FDA's regulatory approach to opioids has consistently failed to adequately protect children from lethal exposures [19]. While some safety measures exist that directly address pediatric risks, significant gaps remain in how these life-threatening drugs are regulated. Moreover, as noted earlier, while the expansion of MAT across the United States has undoubtedly saved many adult lives, because treatment programs rarely incorporate family safety planning or education into their treatment protocols, children continue to be harmed.

Over the years, I have seen rising pediatric exposures to methadone and buprenorphine concurrent with the expansion of these treatment programs. In an effort to quell the cravings associated with opioid withdrawal, essentially one opioid is being substituted for another. These medications have been life-saving for adults and are critically important, but they remain a largely unrecognized threat to children. The same is true for long-acting opioids that are prescribed for chronic pain, like fentanyl patches, which are especially lethal to children even in minimal doses. Because of the chemical makeup of long-acting opioids, they are especially dangerous for children and can cause respiratory depression or death.

Unfortunately, my research has revealed that a disproportionate number of children die from methadone, Suboxone, and fentanyl (Duragesic) pain patches. In the mortality study referenced in Chap. 4, I found that prescription opioids were implicated in 73% of all pediatric opioid deaths, with methadone alone accounting for one-third of deaths across the entire 18-year study period. It is important to note that pediatric deaths from methadone peaked in 2007 and declined steadily thereafter, largely due to an FDA Public Health Advisory (black box warning) alerting clinicians of the risks associated with using methadone for pain management in the adult population [20, 21].

Since then, the DEA and methadone manufacturers have limited the distribution of the highest formulations of the drug (i.e., 40 mg tablets) to hospitals and facilities with MAT programs. While this regulatory action led to a reduction in pediatric methadone poisonings beginning in 2007, Lovegrove et al. noted that poisonings from buprenorphine began to rise around this time [22, 23]. More than 11,000 calls were made to US poison control centers for pediatric buprenorphine exposures between 2007 and 2016; nearly 90% were among children younger than age 6 [24].

5.7 The Unintended Consequence of Changes to Methadone Policy During COVID

While the 2007 FDA black box warnings successfully limited the distribution of methadone, more recent policy changes have undermined these protections and inadvertently brought methadone into thousands of homes that contain children. Prior to the COVID pandemic, methadone patients were typically required to visit clinics daily to receive their doses under supervision. *This restrictive approach, while burdensome for patients, kept the drug out of homes where children might access it*. When COVID arrived, emergency measures allowed clinics to provide 14 to 28 days of take-home doses with minimal oversight regarding home storage. While these changes made treatment more accessible for adults, they introduced potent opioids into thousands of homes without corresponding safety requirements.

This policy shift exemplifies how even well-intentioned measures to help adults with opioid use disorder can inadvertently increase the risks to children when family safety is not considered. When these restrictions were loosened, concurrent safety measures should have addressed how methadone would be packaged and stored within homes. After all, the original clinic-based restrictions existed precisely because unsupervised access posed too high a risk for abuse, diversion (e.g., nonmedical use or selling the drug on the street), and overdose.

The COVID era changes illustrate the lack of consideration that has been given to children when making opioid policy decisions. Policymakers focused on maintaining adult treatment access failed to consider the safety implications for any children living in the homes of those prescribed methadone. A comprehensive approach would have recognized that increasing methadone accessibility required the implementation of simultaneous safeguards to protect children—addressing both adult treatment needs and pediatric safety concerns concurrently.

5.8 Practices That Prioritize Adults Over Children

The practice and policy failures we see in terms of protecting children from opioid poisonings can also be seen in the policies designed to protect infants exposed in utero to opioids. Despite the innovative programs like the Eat, Sleep, Console approach that have emerged in recent years to address the NOWS epidemic, the overall approach in the United States to the public health crisis resulting from newborn exposure to substances in utero prioritizes the needs of adults with substance use disorders over those of their children. For adults, the trend in recent years has been to move away from practices that are considered stigmatizing, punitive, or coercive. Perhaps the best example of this is efforts by states to limit toxicology testing in newborns without parents' consent when substance exposure is suspected. Because of this movement away from toxicology testing, it is not currently known how many infants are exposed in utero to substances. Prior to the opioid crisis, researchers estimated that more than 400,000 children were exposed annually to drugs or alcohol prenatally [25]. This number is almost certainly higher today given the dramatic rise in opioid use among women of childbearing age in recent years.

Even if it is determined that an infant has been exposed in utero, doctors may be discouraged from alerting CPS. In many states, substance exposure is considered insufficient for establishing a CPS report. In large measure this is because many feel that CPS is not only ineffective at addressing the needs of families affected by substance use but also because CPS involvement creates a harmful cycle: parents who are stigmatized and fear losing their children may avoid seeking healthcare, which can lead to worse outcomes for both the mother and the child.

5.9 Child Protection Policies: The Inadequacy of Plans of Safe Care

Within our child protection system, a safety plan refers to the Child Abuse Prevention and Treatment Act (CAPTA) Plan of Safe Care—often referred to as a safety plan or family care plan. CAPTA is a federal law that was enacted in 1974 with the intent to address child abuse and neglect through policy and the provision of federal funding [26]. For nearly 30 years, the legislation did not address infants exposed in utero to drugs or alcohol, but revisions to the law over the past two decades have required states to notify DCF (or CPS, as it is known in certain states) when a child has been exposed to drugs or alcohol in utero. States are also required to develop "plans of safe care" (POSC) for infants exposed to illegal substances or diagnosed with fetal alcohol syndrome or drug withdrawal. Because of the growing opioid crisis, the 2016 Comprehensive Addiction and Recovery Act—also federal law—expanded CAPTA to include infants withdrawing from prescription opioids and clarified that the family care plans (i.e., also referred to as family recovery plans or safety plans) should address the needs of both infants and their caregivers.

States have taken various measures to comply with CAPTA law, with some developing an electronic portal to notify the state's welfare agency that a child has been exposed and a POSC developed. For example, in Connecticut, a CAPTA notification portal was put into effect in 2019. All hospitals in the state are required to submit a notification when an infant is born with prenatal drug/alcohol exposure. In Connecticut, the portal is managed by DCF, and the notification is "blind," meaning that no identifying information is entered for either the child or for the parents. While a family care plan must accompany the report, DCF does not become involved unless the healthcare provider suspects abuse or neglect. Currently, there are efforts underway to make de-identified CAPTA notifications national policy.

5.10 Healthcare Provider Knowledge Gaps and Displacement of Responsibility

The inadequate protections for children evident in POSC are mirrored in the approach healthcare providers take toward opioid safety. While providers serve as a primary source of information for families, I have found, in my research interviewing healthcare providers who routinely care for newborns with NOWS or their mothers, troubling gaps in knowledge and confusion about who is responsible for educating families about opioid safety.

Over several years, I interviewed a wide range of providers involved in maternal and infant care. Strikingly, very few providers were responsible for both mother and baby; primarily social workers bridge this gap. When I asked providers about whether they talked to families about opioid safety (storage, disposal, naloxone use), most acknowledged the importance of such education but did not feel it was their role to deliver it. Many believed that these conversations should be postponed until the child was older and mobile (crawling, walking). As one provider responsible for discharging new mothers and their newborns home from the hospitalization explained: "I'm thinking it's a newborn. It's five days old. It's not going to get into anything. That might be something to certainly think about as they become toddlers for sure." Another provider echoed this sentiment: "I would hope that the pediatrician who is working with the family over those many months and years would have those conversations. To me, my first impression, it would be really, really early to have a discussion about what you would do in ten months or a year or more."

These responses reveal dangerous misconceptions about when children face risks from opioids. Research shows that infants are among the most vulnerable groups, and numerous fatalities have occurred among infants due to exposure from opioid residue on surfaces (including bedding) or transdermal contact with medication patches. There is also documented evidence of parents administering opioids, such as methadone, to infants to calm them or induce sleep—a practice that can prove fatal. Additionally, many providers fail to recognize that the postpartum period represents a time of heightened overdose risk for mothers with opioid use disorder.

Beyond knowledge gaps, many providers express discomfort with initiating conversations about substance use, as many were never trained to do so. As one provider stated: "I think sometimes people are reticent to have those kind of very direct conversations because they're feeling like maybe they are stigmatizing, accusing people. It's just that those challenging conversations need to be had, and I think they can be had in a respectful manner that isn't accusatory." This discomfort creates yet another barrier to effective family education surrounding opioids.

Perhaps most concerning is that even emergency first responders often lack knowledge about naloxone use for pediatric patients [27]. Through my work, I have heard or read of numerous cases where first responders hesitated or failed to administer naloxone to young children due to misunderstandings about the appropriateness of naloxone safety for young children, particularly when the child is an infant.

The fragmentation of the US healthcare system clearly compounds these issues. When everyone assumes that it is the responsibility of another provider to talk to families about opioid safety, these crucial conversations simply fail to happen. This systemic gap in provider knowledge and accountability represents one of the most significant missed opportunities in our response to the opioid crisis.

5.11 Emergency Preparedness and Public Health Messaging

Beyond the gaps in provider knowledge are equally concerning failures in broader public health education and emergency preparedness. Few families have been educated about how to recognize the signs of opioid intoxication. Fewer still have been taught how to respond if a child is poisoned or an adult overdoses. In my research examining the circumstances surrounding fatal pediatric opioid poisonings, I found that parents rarely initiated Cardiopulmonary Resuscitation (CPR), contacted Poison Control, or administered naloxone [9].

Addressing these gaps is critical. The opioid epidemic has been conceptualized as an adult problem rather than a public health risk to children and families. Even among states with strong public health initiatives about protecting communities from opioids, the messaging rarely addresses children. In Wisconsin, for example, the Dose of Reality initiative represents a comprehensive public health campaign that aims to educate communities about opioid dangers—yet even this well-designed program focuses only on adults [28].

The website includes a page that addresses opioid overdose and explains in detail how to recognize the signs: unresponsiveness, slowed or stopped respirations, snoring or rattling breaths, cold or clammy skin, and discoloration of the extremities (cyanosis) that reflects lack of oxygen. The website describes specific steps to take in response to these signs of overdose, such as calling 911, beginning CPR, or giving naloxone. This is essential information, but it focuses only on adult overdoses and not the signs to look for in children [29].

The fundamental problem is that most families have not been taught about the dangers of opioids. This represents a major failure on the part of the medical establishment. Families have not been educated to understand that opioids should be treated with the same caution routinely applied to other household hazards, such as cleaning products, chemicals, knives, and weapons. Opioids are routinely left in unlocked medicine cabinets or out in the open where a child can easily access them. For a small child, even a tiny exposure can be lethal. The failure to help families understand the dangers that opioids pose to children reflects broad societal issues that can only be addressed through comprehensive education that helps families understand the systemic nature of the crisis, namely, adults don't use opioids in isolation but in the context of their families, putting everyone at risk unless safeguards are implemented.

The scale of the problem becomes clear when examining the pediatric exposure data. A 2017 study published in the journal *Pediatrics* by Allen et al. reported that 32 calls are made to poison control centers across the United States every day for opioid poisonings in children [30]. Given that the pediatric opioid crisis has worsened substantially since this study was published, the number of calls to poison control centers is almost certainly higher now. Regardless, the findings from this study remain relevant today. The researchers found that between 2000 and 2015, there were 188,468 opioid exposures in children and adolescents younger than 20 years of age. During this 16-year period, nearly 60% of the exposures were among children younger than 6 years of age, and buprenorphine, one of the primary drugs used as part of MAT for opioid use disorder, led to a disproportionate number of poisonings. Eighty-eight percent of buprenorphine exposures were in young children, and nearly one-half required hospital admission.

In a more recent analysis, researchers found that most opioid exposures in children are from prescription drugs that belong to their parents, grandparents, or other family members [3]. Children were frequently exposed to already opened medication bottles, divided pills and sublingual film strips, discarded fentanyl (e.g., Duragesic) pain patches, and opioid residue left on cotton balls and tissue paper.

5.12 Multi-level Prevention Strategies

The patterns revealed in my research on fatal pediatric opioid poisonings point to several critical opportunities for intervention that our current healthcare system has largely overlooked. First, healthcare providers who prescribe opioids to adults, whether for pain management or opioid use disorder, must integrate family safety planning into standard practice. My finding that nearly 40% of pediatric opioid fatalities occur in the child's own home underscores the urgency of this approach [2]. While many prescribers discuss medication side effect with patients, few discuss secure storage methods or the specific risks these medications pose to children in the household.

Second, the substantial overlap between substance use and child maltreatment documented across all pediatric age groups calls for integrated service models. Child welfare agencies and substance use treatment providers typically operate in separate systems with minimal coordination. Comprehensive family-centered care that simultaneously addresses parental substance use and child safety could prevent many tragic deaths. That 45% of children aged 0 to 4 who died from an opioid poisoning had a caregiver with a history of substance use points to this critical opportunity for intervention [9].

Third, the finding that 42% of children aged 10 to 14 who died from opioid poisoning had their own history of substance use raises an urgent need for earlier screening and intervention with younger adolescents. This age group has been largely overlooked in prevention efforts, with most initiatives targeting older teens. School-based screening programs and pediatric primary care settings represent underutilized venues for identifying substance use in this vulnerable age group.

Finally, universal naloxone distribution should prioritize high-risk families—particularly those with histories of maltreatment and substance use. However, it is important for families to understand that they cannot rely on naloxone alone, as it will not reverse the effects of nonopioid substances [1, 2, 9]. I found, for example, in my analysis of deaths from fentanyl that benzodiazepines were implicated in 17% of fatalities, cocaine in 12%, psychostimulants in 10%, and alcohol in 6% [1]. These findings underscore why families need comprehensive emergency response education that goes beyond naloxone administration to include recognition of poisoning symptoms in children, knowing when to seek emergency care, and age-appropriate resuscitation techniques. Critically, parents must understand that even when naloxone appears effective, emergency medical care is imperative to ensure that the child is medically stable.

The urgent need for comprehensive family education became particularly clear during the COVID pandemic. This public health crisis disrupted the external systems that normally serve to protect children and families. In my recent analysis of national mortality data, I found that fentanyl deaths peaked in 2020 and 2021, suggesting that COVID likely exacerbated the pediatric opioid crisis [1]. With school closures and stay-at-home orders, children spent more time at home and, thus, were more likely to be exposed to parental opioids, while losing the protective factors of school-based supervision.

5.13 Research and Surveillance: Gaps in Knowledge

Our national response to the pediatric opioid crisis has been hampered by the severe limitations that exist in how we track, measure, and learn from the tragic deaths of children. Death certificate data show that at least 15,000 children have died from opioid poisoning over the past three decades. The true toll is certainly much higher. We simply do not have systems in place to capture the full scope of the pediatric opioid crisis.

Because of the inherent difficulty of determining cause of death for any individual—whether for a child or an adult—we do not have a reliable estimate of how many children have died from opioids. Determining cause of death in a child is complicated by multiple factors, including variations across states in how deaths among children are investigated and reported [31, 32]. Better data are needed to understand both the depth and breadth of the opioid crisis and its impact on children. Our inability to fully understand and address pediatric opioid fatalities is further complicated by the common dismissal of these deaths as rare events, especially when compared to adult fatalities. This dismissal in turn justifies limited investment and prioritization of resources.

As Dr. Emily Putnam-Hornstein, a professor at the School of Social Work at the University of North Carolina at Chapel Hill, and Dr. Sarah Font, an associate professor of sociology and public policy at Penn State University, aptly note in a recent article regarding child maltreatment deaths:

> Even if one considers one death to be a numerically rare outcome of child abuse and neglect, that is hardly a reason not to study the incidents that occur and make serious efforts to prevent them. Any number of rare but severe events have led to meaningful changes in social policy because it is unjustifiable to allow them to persist if they can be prevented… Perhaps they are better understood as a canary in the coal mine—a sign of poor or deteriorating standards identifying and responding to children at risk of serious harm.

Our surveillance infrastructure for investigating pediatric opioid deaths exemplifies these "poor standards" [31]. Child Death Review (CDR) teams exist in all states to investigate child fatalities, but their approaches vary widely across the United States. Some states investigate only deaths deemed suspicious, while others examine all child deaths—natural, accidental, homicides, and undetermined [32]. While the National Center for Fatality Review and Prevention was established in 2002 to serve as a central database for CDRs, only 43 states contribute data to the system, and just 24 states legally mandate annual reporting. The quality and consistency of the data reported are often poor, which limits their utility for driving changes to clinical practice and policy initiatives.

I have seen this firsthand in my research examining the circumstances surrounding deaths in children from opioids. After years of cleaning and coding data on approximately 1700 children who died from opioid poisonings between 2004 and 2020, I found that more than 90% of critical data—like how opioids were stored, whether they came in child-resistant packaging, and whether parents administered CPR or naloxone—were missing. Without comprehensive data on the circumstances of pediatric opioid fatalities—including the source of the opioids, the storage methods employed, and the family risk factors—we cannot design effective prevention strategies [9].

Despite the limitations of our surveillance systems, one critical insight emerges from the available data—whether from CDC death certificate data or records gathered by CDR teams: children are dying from opioids primarily at home. This finding represents perhaps the most important discovery from my research over the past 15 years. Nearly 40% of children died in their own homes, and over 60% died outside of any medical setting [6]. This fundamental insight represents a crucial starting point for rethinking our approach to prevention. When we accept that the home environment is where the opioid crisis primarily unfolds, we can redirect our focus from complex institutional solutions toward practical, family-centered interventions.

Yet, more than 30 years into this crisis, most families in the United States still do not have a basic understanding of the risks that opioids pose to themselves or their families. This is a systemic failure on the part of the government and healthcare providers to educate families about opioids and to help them implement common-sense measures that would undoubtedly lead to fewer opioid exposures for both children and adults. As a consequence, research shows that when a poisoning does occur, most families fail to call Poison Control or administer CPR [9]. These are basic emergency response measures that often mean the difference between life and death.

References

1. Gaither JR. National trends in pediatric deaths from Fentanyl, 1999–2021. JAMA Pediatr. 2023; https://doi.org/10.1001/jamapediatrics.2023.0793.
2. Gaither JR, Shabanova V, Leventhal JM. US national trends in pediatric deaths from prescription and illicit opioids, 1999–2016. JAMA Netw Open. 2018;1(8):e186558. https://doi.org/10.1001/jamanetworkopen.2018.6558.
3. Rosen PE, Greller HA, Ramdin C, Ruck B, Nelson LS, Calello DP. Preventing pediatric opioid poisoning: unusual sources and scenarios. J Pediatr. 2024;275:114236. https://doi.org/10.1016/j.jpeds.2024.114236.
4. Grissinger M. Fentanyl transdermal patches: more protection needed for patients and families. https://pmc.ncbi.nlm.nih.gov/articles/PMC2799102/#:~:text=Fentanyl%20patches%20for%20use%20at,seeing%20them%20apply%20a%20patch. Accessed 20 Aug 2025.
5. Lavonas EJ, Banner W, Bradt P, et al. Root causes, clinical effects, and outcomes of unintentional exposures to buprenorphine by young children. J Pediatr. 2013;163(5):1377–83 e1-3. https://doi.org/10.1016/j.jpeds.2013.06.058.
6. Gaither JR, Leventhal JM, Ryan SA, Camenga DR. National trends in hospitalizations for opioid poisonings among children and adolescents, 1997 to 2012. JAMA Pediatr. 2016;170(12):1195–201. https://doi.org/10.1001/jamapediatrics.2016.2154.
7. Gaither JR. The impact of the opioid crisis on neonates, children, and adolescents. In: Suresh S, Shah R, editors. Opioid therapy in children and adolescents. 1st ed. Springer Science; 2020. p. 17–30.
8. Gaither JR, Drago MJ, Grossman MR, et al. Hospital readmissions among infants with neonatal opioid withdrawal syndrome. JAMA Netw Open. 2024;7(9):e2435074. https://doi.org/10.1001/jamanetworkopen.2024.35074.

9. Gaither JR, McCollum S, Bechtel K, Leventhal JM, Mintz S. The circumstances surrounding fatal pediatric opioid poisonings, 2004–2020. Pediatrics. 2024;154(Suppl 3). https://doi.org/10.1542/peds.2024-067043N.
10. Guy GP Jr, Zhang K, Bohm MK, et al. Vital signs: changes in opioid prescribing in the United States, 2006–2015. MMWR Morb Mortal Wkly Rep. 2017;66(26):697–704. https://doi.org/10.15585/mmwr.mm6626a4.
11. Dart RC, Surratt HL, Cicero TJ, et al. Trends in opioid analgesic abuse and mortality in the United States. N Engl J Med. 2015;372(3):241–8. https://doi.org/10.1056/NEJMsa1406143.
12. Centers for Disease Control and Prevention. Opioid Dispensing Rate Map. https://www.cdc.gov/overdose-prevention/data-research/facts-stats/opioid-dispensing-rate-maps.html. Accessed 13 Aug 2025.
13. Gaither JR, Goulet JL, Becker WC, et al. Guideline-concordant management of opioid therapy among Human Immunodeficiency Virus (HIV)-infected and uninfected veterans. J Pain. 2014;15(11):1130–40. https://doi.org/10.1016/j.jpain.2014.08.004.
14. Gaither JR, Goulet JL, Becker WC, et al. The association between receipt of guideline-concordant long-term opioid therapy and all-cause mortality. J Gen Intern Med. 2016;31(5):492–501. https://doi.org/10.1007/s11606-015-3571-4.
15. American Pain Society/American Academy of Pain Medicine. The use of opioids for treatment of chronic pain. A consensus statement from the American Academy of Pain Medicine and the American Pain Society. Clin J Pain. 1997;13:6–8.
16. Chou R, Fanciullo GJ, Fine PG, et al. Clinical guidelines for the use of chronic opioid therapy in chronic noncancer pain. J Pain. 2009;2:113–30.
17. Gaither JR, Goulet JL, Becker WC, et al. The effect of substance use disorders on the association between guideline-concordant long-term opioid therapy and all-cause mortality. J Addict Med. 2016;10(6):418–28. https://doi.org/10.1097/ADM.0000000000000255.
18. Gaither JR, Gordon K, Crystal S, et al. Racial disparities in discontinuation of long-term opioid therapy following illicit drug use among black and white patients. Drug Alcohol Depend. 2018;192:371–6. https://doi.org/10.1016/j.drugalcdep.2018.05.033.
19. Kolodny A. How FDA failures contributed to the opioid crisis. AMA J Ethics. 2020;22(1):E743–50. https://doi.org/10.1001/amajethics.2020.743.
20. Centers for Disease Control and Prevention. Risk for overdose from methadone used for pain relief – United States, 1999–2010. Vital signs factsheet 2012. https://www.cdc.gov/mmwr/preview/mmwrhtml/mm6126a5.htm. Accessed 7 June 2016.
21. Jones CM, Baldwin GT, Manocchio T, White JO, Mack KA. Trends in methadone distribution for pain treatment, methadone diversion, and overdose deaths – United States, 2002–2014. MMWR Morb Mortal Wkly Rep. 2016;65(26):667–71. https://doi.org/10.15585/mmwr.mm6526a2.
22. Lovegrove MC, Mathew J, Hampp C, Governale L, Wysowski DK, Budnitz DS. Emergency hospitalizations for unsupervised prescription medication ingestions by young children. Pediatrics. 2014;134(4):e1009–16. https://doi.org/10.1542/peds.2014-0840.
23. Lovegrove MC, Weidle NJ, Budnitz DS. Trends in emergency department visits for unsupervised pediatric medication exposures, 2004–2013. Pediatrics. 2015;136(4):e821–9. https://doi.org/10.1542/peds.2015-2092.
24. American Association of Poison Control Centers. Opioid (Narcotic) Pain Medications. http://www.aapcc.org/alerts/opioids/. Accessed 23 Feb 2017.
25. National Center on Substance A, Child W, United States. Substance A, Mental Health Services A, United States. Administration for C, Families. Substance-exposed infants: state responses to the problem. HHS publication no (SMA) 09-4369. U.S. Department of Health and Human Services, Substance Abuse and Mental Health Services Administration; 2009.
26. Sieger MHL, Nichols C, Chasnoff IJ. Child Abuse Prevention and Treatment Act, family care plans and infants with prenatal substance exposure: theoretical framework and directions for future research. Infant Child Dev. 2022;31(3). https://doi.org/10.1002/icd.2309.
27. Children's Hospital of Philadelphia. Naloxone is going "over the counter": will it reach our kids? https://policylab.chop.edu/blog/naloxone-going-over-counter-will-it-reach-our-kids. Accessed 20 Aug 2025.

28. Wisconsin Department of Health Services. Dose of reality: opioids in Wisconsin. https://www.dhs.wisconsin.gov/opioids/index.htm. Accessed 24 Sept 2024.
29. Wisconsin Department of Health Services. Dose of reality: opioid overdose. https://www.dhs.wisconsin.gov/opioids/overdose.htm. Accessed 20 Aug 2025.
30. Allen JD, Casavant MJ, Spiller HA, Chounthirath T, Hodges NL, Smith GA. Prescription opioid exposures among children and adolescents in the United States: 2000–2015. Pediatrics. 2017;139(4). https://doi.org/10.1542/peds.2016-3382.
31. Putnam-Hornstein EFS. Why is national child welfare leadership silent on child deaths? https://imprintnews.org/opinion/why-is-national-child-welfare-leadership-silent-on-child-deaths/252134. Accessed 18 Jan 2025.
32. The National Center for the Review and Prevention of Child Deaths. CDR process. https://ncfrp.org/cdr/cdr-process/. Accessed 29 Feb 2024.

6

Ground Zero: Learning to Live with Opioids in Our Homes and Communities

In this chapter, I outline a family-focused, child-centered framework for living safely with opioids in our homes and communities, the primary settings where opioid exposures and fatalities occur. Drawing upon foundational principles of child safety, this comprehensive approach reduces the risk for everyone in the household—children and adults alike. The framework I propose offers concrete guidance across three critical domains: family education, provider support, and pragmatic safety measures. Families need specific knowledge about identifying opioids, recognizing drug toxicity, implementing commonsense safety measures, and responding to emergencies. Healthcare providers need practical strategies for communicating vital safety information during key clinical encounters. Most importantly, this chapter provides details on accessible safety measures—secure storage through lockboxes, systematic disposal via community programs, and comprehensive emergency preparedness with naloxone—that substantially mitigate risks. While these immediate interventions empower families to protect themselves today, broader systemic reforms remain essential to address the root causes of this devastating crisis

6.1 A Family-Focused Framework

As established in Chap. 4, research shows that children and adults face the greatest vulnerability to opioids in the places where they should feel the safest: their homes. Across all ages, this is where most opioid exposures occur and most fatalities happen. Yet, it is in the home that families are least prepared to manage these risks. Through a family-focused, child-centered framework, we can equip families with the knowledge, tools, and resources they need to protect themselves and create safer homes.

6.2 A Child-Centered Approach That Benefits Everyone

My overarching philosophy is both simple and evidence-based: when we design safety systems with children in mind, we extend protections to everyone in the household. Throughout history, our society has successfully helped parents mitigate countless household hazards—from securing cleaning products to removing excess bedding from a child's crib—yet we have failed to apply this same level of pragmatic, commonsense thinking to opioids. By framing opioid safety as a family concern rather than a societal addiction issue, we remove unnecessary stigma and provide families with a sense of control they often lack. This sense of agency is particularly important in the context of addiction, which often leaves families overwhelmed by chaos, hopelessness, and despair—even for family members who themselves do not struggle with substance use.

Importantly, the measures proposed in this chapter apply universally to all families—not just to those affected by substance use. As discussed in Chap. 5, many pediatric opioid poisonings occur in households where opioids were prescribed to manage pain or treat addiction. Creating universal opioid safety standards acknowledges that opioids, whether obtained illicitly or prescribed for pain management or addiction treatment, require the same level of caution and protection we routinely apply to other potential household dangers.

6.3 Education: What Families Need to Know

For effective protection, families and their healthcare providers must first recognize the serious risks that opioids pose within the home environment. Three decades into this crisis, most parents—and surprisingly, many clinicians—lack a fundamental understanding of opioids' dangers to children.

Over the past 2 years, as part of my research aimed at understanding what parents know about opioids, I have conducted interviews with mothers who have delivered infants with NOWS. This work has revealed alarming gaps in knowledge: few mothers understand the potency of these drugs, how rapidly they can suppress a child's breathing, or how even microscopic exposures can prove fatal. These gaps in understanding leave families vulnerable, a vulnerability that is compounded when the family is also struggling with the complexities of substance use, chronic pain, or caring for an ill newborn.

Comprehensive education for families should encompass several critical domains. First, families need a higher degree of medical literacy when it comes to opioids. Patients often fail to recognize that they have been prescribed opioids. Moreover, in my work interviewing families, I've learned that most parents do not realize that drugs like hydrocodone, codeine, methadone, buprenorphine (including Suboxone), and the Duragesic patch (fentanyl) all belong to the same drug class, let alone understand their potency or risk profiles. Without this basic knowledge, parents cannot adequately assess risks. Parents may take great care to secure prescription pain medications but leave drugs prescribed as part of MAT out in the open, not realizing that both pose similar dangers to children. The lack of adequate prescription labeling for opioids further complicates this issue and underscores the important role that healthcare providers and pharmacists play in educating families.

Second, families need practical knowledge about how to recognize the signs of opioid toxicity. Parents should know to look for excessive sleepiness, pinpoint pupils, slowed breathing, blue lips or fingernails (cyanosis), and difficulty walking or talking. Early recognition of these warning signs is especially important when it comes to pediatric opioid exposures—where a delay of minutes could be fatal.

Third, education must address emergency response procedures. Families should know the exact sequence of steps to take if a poisoning or overdose is suspected: call 911 immediately; administer naloxone, if available; begin CPR or rescue breathing, if the child is unresponsive; and contact their state poison control center for additional guidance. Parents must understand that the order matters and minutes count—respiratory depression can rapidly lead to brain damage or death, especially in small children. Because parents may hesitate to use naloxone on their children, education must emphasize that naloxone is safe for anyone of any age, even infants, and that it causes no harm even if the child did not actually ingest opioids.

Finally, parental education should address the misconceptions that often prevent families from implementing safety measures. Parents may feel that their child is too young to come into contact with opioids or that their teen would never experiment with prescription or illicit drugs. Many families also assume that they are immune to the opioid crisis, viewing it as a problem that is relevant only to "other" families, particularly those affected by substance use. These misconceptions increase a family's vulnerability. Babies who are not yet crawling can still be exposed to opioids through residue on bedding or other surfaces, including from transdermal pain patches. Adolescents, regardless of their background, remain vulnerable to experimentation and peer pressure. These misconceptions leave families unprepared to manage the very real risks that opioids pose to children of all ages and across all backgrounds. This is a universal issue, not one limited to certain groups or communities.

Healthcare providers are uniquely positioned to deliver opioid education at multiple points in their contact with families, including during pediatric well-child visits, routine medical appointments, and pharmacy visits when opioid prescriptions are dispensed. Yet, research shows that these conversations rarely happen and opportunities to educate families are too often missed.

6.4 Enhancing Provider Education to Support Families

Healthcare providers need specific training to effectively educate families about opioid safety, including general education about opioids and their effects on families, as well as education that addresses the specific risks opioids pose to children at different ages. Provider education should address how to skillfully communicate with families who are struggling with substance use. This content should be incorporated widely into the curricula of medical and nursing programs, and continuing education should require that healthcare providers stay up to date on emerging threats from opioids and other substances.

Providers across specialties must understand the risks that opioids pose to families as well as the age-specific risks. For instance, providers must understand that babies can be fatally exposed to opioids even if they are not yet crawling or walking. Numerous infants have died after coming into contact with drug residue or medication patches. Similarly, providers, including first responders, should be educated about the appropriateness of naloxone for children of all ages—even infants.

Communication training is equally important. Providers need specific training in how to communicate effectively with families about substance use in a nonstigmatizing manner [1, 2]. While significant effort has gone into reducing stigmatizing language toward families affected by substance use, including initiatives by the American Academy of Pediatrics (AAP) [1], my research shows that it remains a substantial problem, particularly among community providers who may not have been exposed to the level of training that is often offered to providers affiliated with academic institutions. This gap reinforces the need to incorporate this type of education into medical and nursing school curricula.

In addition to standardizing the content of opioid education, institutional protocols should clearly identify which providers are responsible for teaching families about opioid safety and at which point of contact within the healthcare system. For instance, Obstetrics and Gynecology (OB-GYN) providers should begin talking to mothers with OUD during prenatal visits about the risks that opioids pose to both them and their children and start a dialogue about keeping naloxone on hand and planning for safe storage of both prescribed and illicit opioids. When newborns with NOWS are discharged, nurses and physicians should provide standardized education that builds on the discharge education families already receive regarding car seats and safe sleep. Pediatricians should incorporate brief safety screenings into well-child visits, asking not just about opioids in the home but also about all drugs, and use these opportunities to address how opioids should be stored and disposed of. Pain management specialists and addiction treatment providers should discuss family safety before prescribing opioids and ensure families understand the particular dangers that long-acting opioids, such as methadone, Suboxone, and the Duragesic fentanyl patch, pose to young children due to their chemical makeup [3]. Equally important is the role that pharmacists should play in reinforcing education about proper storage and disposal of opioids.

While there are few successful models for integrating opioid safety into standard healthcare protocols, some promising approaches are emerging. For instance, the MOMs (Maternal Overdose Matters) Project in Colorado is an initiative that provides overdose education and naloxone distribution directly to at-risk mothers during their hospital-based labor and delivery stay [4, 5]. Building on this model, I am currently developing the KIDOs (Kids In Danger of Opioids) initiative at Yale-New Haven Hospital in Connecticut, which will implement a "meds to beds" approach to provide opioid education and naloxone training to mothers of infants with NOWS prior to hospital discharge [6]. Mothers will view a brief video about opioid safety and naloxone administration and also receive a lockbox for opioid storage. By embedding this type of safety education into routine care, these programs normalize safety education and reduce associated stigma. Similar protocols should be adapted for emergency departments, primary care settings, and community health centers across the country.

These targeted initiatives align with broader policy shifts recognizing the need for family-focused approaches. In September 2024, the AAP, as part of its guidance to physicians on their role in preventing pediatric poisonings and overdoses, recommended that naloxone be made available to all families regardless of substance use risk [7]. The AAP also recommended that naloxone be routinely prescribed alongside opioid prescriptions [8].

The AAP recognizes that healthcare providers are uniquely positioned to help families navigate the opioid crisis and protect themselves. This is particularly true in the field of pediatrics where pediatricians, nurses, and pharmacists have a well-established culture of educating families about safety and primary prevention [7]. Yet, during the opioid epidemic, many providers—particularly those not directly involved in opioid prescribing—have failed to understand that they have a role to play in protecting children from opioid exposures. As a result, they have missed critical opportunities to educate and support families. Currently, most opioid prescribers fail to routinely ask patients whether they have children in the home. This simple question could trigger a conversation about the risks that opioids pose to children and the commonsense measures that would ensure their safety.

Likewise, pharmacists rarely talk to families about opioid risks even though they interact with families at a critical point—when medications are dispensed. An effective approach is to embed opioid safety into routine care. For example, with every opioid prescription dispensed, pharmacists should include a coprescription for naloxone, as recommended by the AAP. The naloxone could be delivered within a lockbox containing educational materials on opioid safety. Lockboxes, in turn, could feature a QR code linking to an instructional video on proper storage, disposal, and emergency response.

This example illustrates just one of the many opportunities that providers have for intervening across healthcare settings. By equipping all providers—from physicians and nurses to pharmacists and social workers—with the knowledge, communication skills, and institutional support needed to have these conversations, we can empower families to implement protective measures within their homes.

6.5   Practical Home-Safety Measures

With education as our foundation, we can now turn to the practical measures that families can implement to create safer homes. Just as families childproof homes for other hazards, they should also establish baseline safety standards for managing opioids—and all other drugs—whether prescribed or illicit. These measures are neither complex nor expensive. They are straightforward approaches that have proven effective in reducing childhood poisonings from other substances. There are at least three essential components to home opioid safety: proper storage, responsible disposal, and emergency preparedness. By implementing these three measures, families can dramatically reduce the risk of an accidental exposure.

Moreover, the circumstances surrounding fatal pediatric opioid poisonings in different age groups suggest the need for tailored prevention approaches. For families with children under the age of 5, where my research shows that 45% of opioid fatalities involve a caregiver with a history of substance use, interventions must focus on secure medication storage, recognition of poisoning symptoms specific to infants and toddlers, and immediate emergency response [9]. For adolescents, particularly the often-overlooked 10–14-year-old age group where I have found that 42% have their own history of substance use, prevention efforts should include early screening in pediatric primary care and school settings.

I also found that for both younger children and older teens, one in four has a history of child maltreatment (i.e., physical abuse or neglect), which points to the need for child welfare systems to incorporate specific opioid safety planning into their standard protocols for families where substance use is identified as a risk factor.

6.5.1 Safe Storage: Barriers to Access

The most fundamental component of opioid safety is preventing access through safe storage of prescription medications and illicit drugs (and any associated drug paraphernalia), which can substantially reduce the likelihood of opioid exposures. While hospitals treat opioids as controlled substances requiring that they be stored under lock and key, in most American homes, even those with small children, this practice is not followed. Research shows that only a small percentage of families store their prescription opioids in a locked location, and an even smaller percentage use dedicated lockboxes, despite their affordability (available online for less than $30). This gap between hospital and home practices becomes clear when examining family behavior. In a 2017 national survey of adults who were prescribed opioids for pain relief, researchers found that *less than one-third of families with young children in the home reported safely storing their medications* [10]. For those with older children, the percentage was even lower at less than 12%. These low rates are concerning given that effective storage solutions need not be complex or expensive. The modest investment in a lockbox is negligible when compared to the potential consequences of leaving opioids unsecured. For most families, a simple lockbox with a combination lock or key will provide sufficient security.

For adults and adolescents who have been prescribed MAT for opioid use disorder, storage is particularly critical. As previously discussed, methadone and buprenorphine can be lethal in small doses due to their chemical makeup and potency. Suboxone (buprenorphine and naloxone) is particularly concerning because of its packaging and sublingual formulation [3]. To achieve proper dosing, patients may not consume the entire sublingual strip but instead break it into pieces. Reports from poison control centers show that the unused portions, which may be left on the counters or dropped on the floor, are a common source of pediatric opioid poisonings [11].

A growing number of community organizations, including the African American Opioid Coalition [12], and healthcare institutions across the country are providing lockboxes to families free of charge. This simple intervention creates a crucial barrier to access for young children, teens, and even adults.

6.5.2 Safe Disposal: Removing Unnecessary Risks from the Home

Equally important to proper storage is the prompt disposal of unused opioids. Many families keep leftover prescription medications in their homes for years, prolonging both the risks these drugs pose and the opportunities for diversion and abuse. Research has shown that two-thirds of patients prescribed opioids after surgery report not using all of their medications [13], and several studies indicate that unused opioids are not disposed of but instead remain in the home in unsecured locations [14]. This is true even when children are present in the home [10].

Even though unused opioids represent a significant household risk, many families are unaware that unused medications should be disposed of promptly and are unfamiliar with where to do so safely. Unfortunately, healthcare providers frequently lack the knowledge to guide families, despite the availability of four main disposal pathways [15].

- *Community Take-Back Programs*: The Drug Enforcement Administration (DEA) sponsors National Prescription Drug Take Back Day events twice yearly, where medications can be dropped off anonymously at designated locations
- *Permanent Drop Boxes*: Many police stations, hospitals, and pharmacies maintain secure drop boxes for prescription medications. These allow for year-round disposal options. The DEA maintains a website ("Every Day is Take Back Day") listing approximately 17,000 locations nationwide
- *Mail-Back Programs*: Some healthcare systems and pharmacies provide prepaid envelopes for mailing unused medications to specialized disposal facilities. These resources are particularly valuable for families with limited mobility or transportation issues, including those in rural areas
- *At-Home Disposal Methods*: When the community options listed above are not available, the FDA recommends that individuals mix their unused medications with unpalatable materials such as coffee grounds, cat litter, or dirt before placing the mixture in a sealed container and disposing of it in the indoor trash. While not ideal, this approach is preferable to leaving medications inside the home. For fentanyl patches, which can still contain a lethal amount of medication after being removed from the skin, the FDA recommends folding the patch with the adhesive sides together and then flushing it down the toilet. The FDA maintains a "flush list" on its website. Fentanyl, buprenorphine, oxycodone, and methadone are on this list because of the extreme dangers these drugs present to children

By removing unnecessary opioids from the home promptly, families substantially reduce the chances that a child will come into contact with the drugs or that teens and adults will use them improperly.

6.5.3 Emergency Preparedness: When Prevention Fails

Despite our best efforts, emergencies will still occur. As with any other drug, children will continue to ingest opioids, making it essential that all families with individuals in the home who use opioids (or when visitors who use opioids are present) have a comprehensive emergency plan that includes recognizing opioid toxicity, calling emergency services, administering naloxone, and beginning CPR. Multiple layers of protection are necessary because of the lethality of opioids.

Naloxone (commonly known by the brand name Narcan) is a critical tool in emergency preparedness. The medication reverses the effects of opioids by blocking opioid receptors in the brain. When administered in time, naloxone can quickly restore normal respirations, typically within 2 to 3 min, in someone whose respirations have slowed or stopped. If breathing is not restored after the first dose, a second dose can be administered.

It is important for families to understand that naloxone is unique among medications in its safety profile—there are no situations where it is harmful to use in an emergency [16, 17]. If naloxone is given to someone who does not have opioids in their system, it has no effect, and it is safe for all ages, including infants and young children.

However, while naloxone is life-saving, families should understand that it is a last line of defense, not a replacement for the prevention measures outlined earlier in this chapter. The enthusiasm for naloxone in the medical community, while warranted and well-intentioned, should not overshadow the importance of other safety measures. Naloxone is undeniably life-saving, but its use means that all other preventive measures have either failed or were not instituted in the first place. Thus, we must continue to advocate for increasing access to naloxone in homes and communities across the United States while simultaneously investing in family education on opioid risks, emergency preparedness, and proper storage and disposal practices—all essential elements for preventing exposures from occurring in the first place.

Families need to understand several key points about naloxone:

- Naloxone should be kept easily accessible and in multiple locations (home, car, purse)
- It should never be stored locked away with opioids or other medications, so as to make it difficult to access during an emergency
- Expiration dates should be checked regularly. Naloxone typically expires 4 years from the manufacture date
- Used or expired doses should be replaced immediately

An effective emergency plan should be written down and shared with all household members and frequent visitors and include the following:

- Recognizing the warning signs of opioid toxicity
- Naloxone storage locations throughout the home
- Instructions for administering the drug
- Basic CPR instructions
- Step-by-step emergency procedures:
  1. Administer naloxone
  2. Call 911
  3. Begin CPR or rescue breathing
  4. Contact Poison Control (1-800-222-1222)

Please note that emergency response protocols may vary as to whether naloxone should be administered first or 911 called [18, 19]; *ideally, they should be done simultaneously if multiple bystanders are present. The key is to act quickly on both fronts.*

By combining proper storage and disposal of opioids with comprehensive emergency preparedness, families can create multiple layers of protection against opioid dangers. This approach recognizes that no single measure is foolproof, but together these prevention and response measures create a home-safety system that significantly reduces the risk of pediatric opioid exposures.

The practical safety measures outlined in this chapter provide families with immediate tools to protect themselves from opioids. While home-based interventions form the foundation of any comprehensive safety approach, they represent only part of the solution. Families should not bear the entire burden of managing risks caused by systemic failures in medication prescribing and packaging, healthcare delivery, and public policy. The next chapter explores how broader systems—from healthcare practices to regulatory frameworks—must evolve to support family efforts and create comprehensive protection. Until these systemic changes occur, however, the straightforward measures described here offer families concrete ways to reduce risk and create safer environments for everyone in the household, adults and children alike.

References

1. Alinsky RH, Hadland SE, Quigley J, Patrick SW, Committee On Substance USE, Prevention. Recommended terminology for substance use disorders in the care of children, adolescents, young adults, and families. Pediatrics. 2022;149(6). https://doi.org/10.1542/peds.2022-057529.
2. Botticelli MP, Koh HK. Changing the language of addiction. JAMA. 2016;316(13):1361–2. https://doi.org/10.1001/jama.2016.11874.
3. Budnitz DS, Lovegrove MC, Sapiano MR, et al. Notes from the field: pediatric emergency department visits for buprenorphine/naloxone ingestion – United States, 2008–2015. MMWR Morb Mortal Wkly Rep. 2016;65(41):1148–9. https://doi.org/10.15585/mmwr.mm6541a5.

4. Johnson A, Swenson KS, Dillner E, et al. Addressing perinatal substance use: a triad approach led by the Colorado perinatal care quality collaborative. J Midwifery Women's Health. 2024;69(4):586–92. https://doi.org/10.1111/jmwh.13615.
5. Colorado Maternal Mental Health Collaborative. Maternal Overdose Matters Plus (MOMs+). https://cpcqc.org/programs/moms-plus/. Accessed 24 Sept 2024.
6. Gaither JR. Yale School of Medicine: KIDs in Danger of Opioids (KIDO) initiative. https://medicine.yale.edu/kids-in-danger-of-opioids/. Accessed 27 Mar 2025.
7. McKnight E, Holland-Hall C. Pediatricians' role in overdose prevention: a call for universal naloxone dispensing. Pediatrics. 2024;154(4). https://doi.org/10.1542/peds.2024-067258.
8. Hadland SE, Agarwal R, Raman SR, et al. Opioid prescribing for acute pain management in children and adolescents in outpatient settings: clinical practice guideline. Pediatrics. 2024; https://doi.org/10.1542/peds.2024-068752.
9. Gaither JR, McCollum S, Bechtel K, Leventhal JM, Mintz S. The circumstances surrounding fatal pediatric opioid poisonings, 2004–2020. Pediatrics. 2024;154(Suppl 3). https://doi.org/10.1542/peds.2024-067043N.
10. McDonald EM, Kennedy-Hendricks A, McGinty EE, Shields WC, Barry CL, Gielen AC. Safe storage of opioid pain relievers among adults living in households with children. Pediatrics. 2017; https://doi.org/10.1542/peds.2016-2161.
11. American Association of Poison Control Centers. Opioid (Narcotic) Pain Medications. http://www.aapcc.org/alerts/opioids/. Accessed 23 Feb 2017.
12. African American Opioid Coalition. Improving wellness of Black families. https://safercommunity.net/aaocmdc/. Accessed 20 Aug 2025.
13. Bates C, Laciak R, Southwick A, Bishoff J. Overprescription of postoperative narcotics: a look at postoperative pain medication delivery, consumption and disposal in urological practice. J Urol. 2011;185(2):551–5. https://doi.org/10.1016/j.juro.2010.09.088.
14. Bicket MC, Long JJ, Pronovost PJ, Alexander GC, Wu CL. Prescription Opioid analgesics commonly unused after surgery: a systematic review. JAMA Surg. 2017;152(11):1066–71. https://doi.org/10.1001/jamasurg.2017.0831.
15. Food and Drug Administration. Disposal of unused medications: what you should know. https://www.fda.gov/drugs/safe-disposal-medicines/disposal-unused-medicines-what-you-should-know. Accessed 1 Mar 2025.
16. U.S. Food and Drug Administration. NARCAN (naloxone hydrochloride) nasal spray. https://www.accessdata.fda.gov/drugsatfda_docs/label/2015/208411lbl.pdf. Accessed 5 Apr 2020.
17. U.S. Food and Drug Administration. Information about naloxone and nalmefene. https://www.fda.gov/drugs/postmarket-drug-safety-information-patients-and-providers/information-about-naloxone-and-nalmefene. Accessed 27 Mar 2025.
18. Centers for Disease Control and Prevention. 5 things to know about naloxone. https://www.cdc.gov/overdose-prevention/reversing-overdose/about-naloxone.html. Accessed 20 Aug 2025.
19. Substance Abuse and Mental Health Services Administration. Opioid overdose prevention toolkit. https://library.samhsa.gov/sites/default/files/five-essential-steps-for-first-responders.pdf. Accessed 20 Aug 2025.

7

Strengthening the Safety Net: Institutional Approaches to Family Protection

This chapter examines how healthcare systems, regulatory frameworks, and community organizations must evolve to support families in protecting themselves from opioids. Building on the home-based interventions described in Chap. 6, we explore systemic approaches that create multiple layers of protection for vulnerable families, beginning with the application of the checklist approach introduced in Chap. 3. Next, we examine how healthcare institutions can embed opioid safety into standard workflows through electronic health record integration and automated safety prompts. Community-based support networks that extend protection beyond clinical settings are also examined, highlighting promising initiatives that provide ongoing family support. Regulatory approaches to medication safety—particularly the successes and limitations of child-resistant packaging—are assessed alongside recommendations for closing critical gaps in current legislation. Finally, emerging models of family-centered addiction treatment that challenge traditional individual-focused paradigms are analyzed, demonstrating how integrated service models address both the needs of parents with substance use disorders and their children. Together, these systemic reforms reinforce and strengthen family-level interventions.

7.1 Beyond Individual Households: Supporting and Reinforcing Family Efforts

While the home-based safety measures outlined in Chap. 6 provide essential protection for families, they represent only part of the solution to America's opioid crisis. Individual families, no matter how vigilant, cannot fully protect themselves without supportive systems, policies, and frameworks that acknowledge the reality of opioids in our communities. The burden of safety should not rest solely on parents and caregivers who are often navigating complex healthcare systems, managing chronic pain, or addressing substance use disorders while also trying to maintain safe homes for their children.

© The Author(s), under exclusive license to Springer Nature Switzerland AG 2026
J. R. Gaither, *Living with Opioids*, https://doi.org/10.1007/978-3-031-95820-5_7

A truly effective approach to opioid safety requires that the healthcare institutions and systems that families encounter in their day-to-day lives actively support their efforts at home. Healthcare providers, pharmacies, addiction treatment centers, child welfare agencies, and regulatory bodies all play critical roles in creating environments where safe practices are reinforced and supported rather than undermined. Applying the child-centered, family-focused principles outlined earlier in this book to these broader systems ensures that we develop approaches that complement and strengthen family efforts rather than leaving families to navigate these challenges alone.

This chapter examines how our institutions and systems must evolve to create multiple layers of protection that extend from clinical settings into communities and homes. We begin by exploring how standardized protocols and simple tools like checklists can transform chaotic, high-stress environments into settings where safety measures are consistently implemented. We then examine specific strategies for how healthcare systems, regulatory frameworks, and community organizations can implement changes that prioritize family safety and well-being.

7.2   A Simple Checklist for a Complex Problem

As discussed in Chap. 3 regarding the care of infants with NOWS, Atul Gawande's checklist approach has transformed safety practices in complex fields like medicine and aviation [1]. This same approach can be applied more broadly to opioid safety across healthcare settings.

Given the complexity and critical importance of ensuring the safety of families affected by opioids, a similar checklist is warranted—particularly during high-stress transitions of care. Discharge planning for families affected by maternal opioid use exemplifies this type of chaotic healthcare environment where critical safety information is easily overlooked. For healthcare workers, caring for a substance-exposed infant is medically intensive, requiring extensive resources and personnel. The discharge planning process is further complicated when DCF is involved, creating a stressful environment where delivering crucial opioid safety information may be overlooked.

A comprehensive checklist for these families would include verification across several important domains:

- Education on opioid identification, risks, and signs of toxicity
- Proper plan for storing opioids in the home
- Disposal plan for unused medications
- Emergency contacts and response plan
- Naloxone availability and knowledge of administration
- Regular safety audits to ensure continued compliance

Successfully implementing such a safety checklist requires coordination among multiple healthcare team members. For infants with NOWS, safety planning should begin at admission and be finalized before discharge.

An effective workflow might involve nursing staff introducing the rationale and need for a safety checklist to families early in the hospitalization and working with them throughout their stay to refine and finalize the document. Social workers would verify that families have access to necessary resources and connect them with community support services. Physicians would review the final safety plan with families, reinforce critical teaching points, and verify that all requirements are met before the family is discharged home. Such a standardized approach should be implemented across all relevant healthcare encounters, making the completion of safety checklists a required element of hospital discharge planning for all families affected by maternal opioid use.

This approach could be adapted across healthcare settings. In primary care, abbreviated versions could be integrated into well-child visits or pain management follow-ups. In emergency departments, modified checklists would be triggered for any patient discharged with an opioid prescription or following an opioid-related visit. Pharmacies could implement similar verification protocols when dispensing opioid medications.

To avoid stigmatization, similar safety checklists could be universally implemented for all families receiving opioid prescriptions, with appropriate modifications based on specific risk factors. This universality normalizes opioid safety as standard practice rather than targeted interventions for "high-risk" families.

The effectiveness of this approach lies in its simplicity and consistency. Rather than expecting providers to remember every safety component during busy clinical encounters, the checklist ensures that essential elements are not missed. When integrated into electronic health records and existing Plans of Safe Care (as mandated by the Child Abuse Prevention and Treatment Act) [2], these checklists can generate automated reminders, track completion across healthcare settings, and promote accountability.

7.3 Healthcare Systems Integration: Embedding Safety at Every Point of Contact

Healthcare systems must move beyond viewing opioid safety as an optional task and recognize it as a core responsibility. This requires integrating safety measures into standardized workflows with clear structures of accountability.

Discharge planning represents a critical opportunity for systems interventions. When patients leave any healthcare setting with an opioid prescription or receive ongoing treatment for an opioid use disorder (such as at methadone clinics), discharge procedures should include the following:

- Provision of lockboxes and naloxone
- Written materials on opioid safety in appropriate languages and literacy levels
- Scheduling follow-up appointments that specifically address medication safety
- Connection to community resources for ongoing support

Electronic health records should be configured to trigger opioid safety protocols whenever relevant medications are prescribed. These automated prompts can serve as clinical decision support rather than merely documentation requirements. Advanced systems can track household prescribing patterns, flagging situations where multiple opioid prescriptions have been issued to the same household.

By embedding these practices into healthcare systems rather than relying on individual provider initiative, we create sustainable change that withstands staff turnover and shifting priorities. Making opioid safety the default path ensures consistency regardless of individual provider preferences or knowledge gaps.

7.4 Evidence-Based Quality of Care and Monitoring

My research on the quality of care received by patients through the VA healthcare system demonstrates the critical importance of structured protocols for monitoring patients. In this examination of more than 20,000 US veterans receiving opioids long term (90 days or more), my colleagues and I found that only 52% of patients received a primary care visit within a month of starting treatment, and only 15% received urine drug testing—both considered basic safety measures [3] according to clinical practice guidelines [4–7].

These findings highlight the need for automated systems that ensure patients prescribed opioids, particularly over long periods, receive appropriate, high-quality care. Electronic health records should be configured to trigger mandatory follow-up appointments, laboratory testing, and risk assessments based on evidence-based guidelines [8]. Such protocols should include the following:

- Required follow-up visits within 1 to 4 weeks of opioid initiation
- Automated ordering of urine drug tests
- Alerts when patients have concurrent sedative prescriptions
- Structured assessments for substance use disorders before and during treatment
- Mandatory documentation of substance use treatment referrals, when indicated

These recommendations align with the CDC's 2022 Clinical Practice Guideline for Prescribing Opioids for Pain, which emphasizes the importance of regular monitoring and careful risk assessment throughout opioid therapy [8].

This research revealed that even veterans, a population that typically has more frequent encounters with the healthcare system [9, 10], still had substantial gaps in safety monitoring [3]. This suggests that even in healthcare systems with regular patient contact, without structured protocols specifically addressing opioid safety, critical follow-up care will be missed.

By embedding these evidence-based guidelines directly into healthcare workflows rather than relying on individual provider initiative, we can ensure that patient safety measures become the default rather than the exception. More broadly, such systems would benefit not only the patients themselves but also protect vulnerable family members, particularly children, from potential exposures to opioids.

7.5 Community-Based Support Networks

Even with improved healthcare approaches, many families need ongoing community support to maintain safe opioid practices. Community-based models that provide such support are emerging across the country.

The MOMs Project in Colorado is an example of a community-based approach that I used as a model for developing the Kids in Danger of Opioids (KIDO) initiative at Yale-New Haven Children's Hospital (detailed in Chap. 5) [11–13]. These programs aim to provide safety education to mothers with opioid use disorder and then connect families to community resources for ongoing support. By embedding opioid education into routine care, these programs normalize safety while reducing stigma.

Similar programs can be expanded to other community settings and populations. Home-visiting nurses and other community healthcare workers are ideally positioned to incorporate comprehensive opioid safety assessments and education into their existing services. Likewise, schools can integrate opioid safety education into existing health curricula and expand school nursing services to include education for families affected by opioid use, distribution of naloxone and lockboxes, and facilitating connections to community resources. Parent-teacher associations could support these outreach efforts. Community organizations focused on substance use treatment and recovery can incorporate opioid safety planning into their peer support services, and churches could host safety workshops and distribute educational materials.

These community-based approaches are particularly important for reaching families who have limited engagement with traditional healthcare systems. By diversifying the messengers and settings for safety education, we increase the likelihood that all families receive the information and safety tools they need.

7.6 Regulatory Approaches: Designing Safety into Products and Systems

Beyond the active safety measures outlined above that require family implementation, we urgently need passive protections engineered directly into opioid products themselves—safety features that automatically safeguard families without requiring any conscious effort on their part.

For opioid medications, we need better product labeling, smaller quantities dispensed per prescription, and, most importantly, child-resistant packaging for all prescription opioids, including those dispensed for opioid use disorder.

Beginning in 1974, child-resistant packaging was required for certain prescription drugs, but not all. This initiative is arguably the single most important contributor to the reduction in childhood poisoning morbidity and mortality from the mid-1970s through the 1990s. During this time, child-resistant packaging resulted in a 45% reduction in pediatric mortality from ingestions of oral prescription drugs

[14]. In 1964, there were approximately 3.5 deaths per million children younger than age 5 [14]. By 1992, deaths from ingestions had dropped to fewer than two deaths per million after the introduction of child-resistant packaging. According to research by G.B. Rodgers published in 1996 on the safety effects of child-resistant packaging, more than 50% of all drug poisonings in children from oral medications involved drugs that were either dispensed in conventional packages (i.e., not child-resistant) or in packaging where the child-resistant feature had been disabled [14].

The public health success of child-resistant packaging demonstrates the power of passive strategies that protect the public. Unlike interventions that require behavior change, passive protections like child-resistant pill bottles do not require any thought on the part of the consumer. Yet, some prescription drugs, including long-acting opioids that are particularly dangerous to children such as *fentanyl pain patches and Suboxone, are still dispensed in packages that provide insufficient barriers to exposure despite containing drugs that have the potency to kill in minuscule amounts* [15–17].

The FDA and the Consumer Product Safety Commission (CPSC) are the main federal agencies responsible for ensuring that drug packaging is safe [18, 19]. The CPSC administers the Poison Prevention Packaging Act (PPPA), significant legislation enacted in 1970 to reduce childhood poisonings from certain household substances (such as cleaning products) and oral prescription medications [20]. This legislation represents one of the most successful passive safety interventions in modern public health history.

Despite the PPPA's success, significant gaps in the legislation have left children vulnerable to opioid exposures. While the act technically requires child-resistant packaging for prescription opioids, several critical exceptions undermine its effectiveness. Prescribers can request non-child-resistant packaging for any patient, and many do so routinely without considering household risks. Additionally, the PPPA was designed primarily for traditional pill bottles, leaving newer formulations like buprenorphine films (dispensed in foil pouches) and *fentanyl patches with packaging that technically complies with regulations but offers minimal protection once opened*. Perhaps most concerning, under PPPA testing protocols, packaging is considered child-resistant if at least 80% of children aged 42 to 51 months cannot open it within a 10-min period [18]. This standard—allowing up to 20% of children to potentially access the contents—may be inadequate for highly potent opioids, like fentanyl, where even a minimal exposure can be fatal to a child.

The PPPA also fails to address medications dispensed from clinics in bulk containers that are then repackaged, a common practice with methadone and other MAT drugs [21]. Take-home doses may be dispensed in containers that meet minimum requirements but are not truly protective given the extreme danger these medications pose to children.

These regulatory gaps in legal, prescribed medications highlight the need for updated standards specifically designed for today's more potent opioid formulations.

7.7 Family-Centered Addiction Treatment and Integrated Models

Beyond regulatory reforms, we also need fundamental changes in how we approach addiction treatment. Despite overwhelming evidence that substance use affects the entire family system [22], addiction treatment in the United States predominantly focuses on the individual with the disorder [23, 24]. The standard approach isolates treatment from the family context, overlooking the parent-child relationship and the needs of children affected by parental substance use—many of whom will struggle throughout their lives with mental health and substance use problems of their own [25–27].

Traditional treatment programs fail to consider the burden that addiction treatment places on the entire family [24]. Parenting responsibilities are rarely considered. Women receiving inpatient treatment or residential treatment are typically separated from their children [28]. For outpatient care, few facilities provide childcare or transportation services [29]. These structural barriers disproportionately affect mothers, who remain the primary caregivers in most families even when struggling with a substance use disorder.

When children's needs are considered, it is usually through separate systems—child welfare agencies or pediatric providers—who operate with minimal coordination with adult treatment providers [30, 31].

Yale University has pioneered several innovative programs including family-based recovery (FBR) [32], which provides in-home services to families with substance use disorders, and other initiatives like Mothering from the Inside Out (MIO) and the Minding the Baby program [33, 34]. These approaches represent a paradigm shift by treating the family unit rather than just the individual with the substance use disorder. For instance, FBR provides home-visiting services to families with young children. Clinicians work with the entire family with the objective of providing substance use treatment in the context of supporting the parent-child relationship. This integrated approach recognizes that strengthening attachment between parents and children can motivate parents to abstain from alcohol and drugs and maintain sobriety.

The Matrix Model for families, developed in Southern California, incorporates family education groups and parent training alongside traditional addiction treatment components [35]. This program recognizes that sustainable recovery requires addressing the parent-child relationship and teaching parenting skills that may have been compromised during active addiction.

Residential programs that accommodate parents and children together represent another promising approach. Facilities like the APT Foundation in Connecticut [36, 37] and Meta House in Wisconsin [38, 39] allow mothers to bring their children into treatment, providing specialized services for both. These programs address parenting challenges in real time, helping mothers develop skills while maintaining crucial attachment relationships with their children.

The expense of these comprehensive approaches represents a significant barrier to wider implementation. Most insurance plans, including Medicaid, provide limited coverage for family therapy and rarely cover supportive services like childcare or parenting education. As a result, family-centered treatment tends to rely on grant funding or philanthropic support [39], creating sustainability challenges and limited availability.

A truly transformative approach would recognize that when a parent struggles with substance use, the entire family needs support. Treatment would routinely include the following:

- Assessment of all family members' needs, including children at different developmental stages
- Parent-child therapy to rebuild attachment and trust
- Practical support like childcare, transportation, and stable housing
- Education about substance use and its impact on children and parenting
- Development of family safety plans that address relapse risks
- Coordination with children's healthcare and educational providers

These family-centered treatment models address one aspect of our fragmented approach to the opioid crisis. However, they can only succeed within a broader system that coordinates care across traditionally siloed services.

The fragmentation of our healthcare systems is perhaps the most fundamental barrier to protecting children from the harms of opioids. Adults and children largely interact with entirely separate systems of care, creating dangerous gaps in communication and coordination. Pediatricians have little understanding of adult substance use and may not even know when parents are prescribed opioids for chronic pain or MAT for opioid use disorders; addiction providers do not screen for or address parenting challenges; and child welfare workers often have different goals and priorities than pediatric and adult healthcare providers.

Building truly integrated systems of care will require fundamental shifts in how we conceptualize and fund services for families affected by substance use. Rather than asking which family member is the "patient," we must recognize that addressing the needs of parents inherently benefits their children, and supporting children strengthens parents' recovery. Chapter 3 outlined how this approach is being implemented for infants with NOWS through models like Eat, Sleep, Console [40–42]; these principles must now be extended throughout our healthcare, addiction treatment, and child welfare systems.

The systemic reforms outlined in this chapter—universal protocols, healthcare integration, community support networks, regulatory changes, and family-centered treatment approaches—represent critical steps toward addressing America's opioid crisis. Implementing these changes will require significant commitment from healthcare institutions, government, and community organizations. In the next chapter, we will look at what can be learned from other nations around the world that have already implemented similar approaches with remarkable success.

References

1. Gawande A. The checklist manifesto: how to get things right. Metropolitan Books; 2010.
2. Sieger MHL, Nichols C, Chasnoff IJ. Child Abuse Prevention and Treatment Act, family care plans and infants with prenatal substance exposure: theoretical framework and directions for future research. Infant Child Dev. 2022;31(3). https://doi.org/10.1002/icd.2309.
3. Gaither JR, Goulet JL, Becker WC, et al. Guideline-concordant management of opioid therapy among human immunodeficiency virus (HIV)-infected and uninfected veterans. J Pain. 2014;15(11):1130–40. https://doi.org/10.1016/j.jpain.2014.08.004.
4. American Pain Society/American Academy of Pain Medicine. The use of opioids for treatment of chronic pain. A consensus statement from the American Academy of Pain Medicine and the American Pain Society. Clin J Pain. 1997;13:6–8.
5. Chou R, Fanciullo GJ, Fine PG, et al. Clinical guidelines for the use of chronic opioid therapy in chronic noncancer pain. J Pain. 2009;2:113–30.
6. Dowell D, Haegerich TM, Chou R. CDC guideline for prescribing opioids for chronic pain – United States, 2016. JAMA. 2016; https://doi.org/10.1001/jama.2016.1464.
7. Dowell D, Ragan KR, Jones CM, Baldwin GT, Chou R. CDC clinical practice guideline for prescribing opioids for pain – United States, 2022. MMWR Recomm Rep. 2022;71(3):1–95. https://doi.org/10.15585/mmwr.rr7103a1.
8. Dowell D, Haegerich TM, Chou R. CDC guideline for prescribing opioids for chronic pain – United States, 2016. MMWR Recomm Rep. 2016;65(1):1–49. https://doi.org/10.15585/mmwr.rr6501e1.
9. Asch SM, Kerr EA, Keesey J, et al. Who is at greatest risk for receiving poor-quality health care? N Engl J Med. 2006;354(11):1147–56. https://doi.org/10.1056/NEJMsa044464.
10. Asch SM, McGlynn EA, Hogan MM, et al. Comparison of quality of care for patients in the Veterans Health Administration and patients in a national sample. Comparative Study. Ann Intern Med. 2004;141(12):938–45.
11. Colorado Maternal Mental Health Collaborative. Maternal Overdose Matters Plus (MOMs+). https://cpcqc.org/programs/moms-plus/. Accessed 24 Sept 2024.
12. Johnson A, Swenson KS, Dillner E, et al. Addressing perinatal substance use: a triad approach led by the Colorado perinatal care quality collaborative. J Midwifery Womens Health. 2024;69(4):586–92. https://doi.org/10.1111/jmwh.13615.
13. Gaither JR. Yale School of Medicine: KIDs in Danger of Opioids (KIDO) initiative. https://medicine.yale.edu/kids-in-danger-of-opioids/. Accessed 27 Mar 2025.
14. Rodgers GB. The safety effects of child-resistant packaging for oral prescription drugs. Two decades of experience. JAMA. 1996;275(21):1661–5.
15. Grissinger M. Fentanyl transdermal patches: more protection needed for patients and families. https://pmc.ncbi.nlm.nih.gov/articles/PMC2799102/#:~:text=Fentanyl%20patches%20for%20use%20at,seeing%20them%20apply%20a%20patch. Accessed 20 Aug 2025.
16. Gaither JR. National trends in pediatric deaths from Fentanyl, 1999–2021. JAMA Pediatr. 2023; https://doi.org/10.1001/jamapediatrics.2023.0793.
17. Lavonas EJ, Banner W, Bradt P, et al. Root causes, clinical effects, and outcomes of unintentional exposures to buprenorphine by young children. J Pediatr. 2013;163(5):1377–83 e1-3. https://doi.org/10.1016/j.jpeds.2013.06.058.
18. United States Consumer Product Safety Commission. Guide to special packaging. https://www.cpsc.gov/Business%2D%2DManufacturing/Business-Education/Business-Guidance/PPPA/Guide-to-Special-Packaging. Accessed 1 Mar 2025.
19. United States Consumer Product Safety Commission. Annual report on pediatric poisoning fatalities and injuries. 2023. Accessed 14 Mar 2024.
20. United States Consumer Product Safety Commission. Poison prevention packaging act business guidance. https://www.cpsc.gov/Business%2D%2DManufacturing/Business-Education/Business-Guidance/PPPA. Accessed 1 Mar 2025.

21. United States Consumer Product Safety Commission. Poison Prevention Packaging Act (PPPA) updated guidance on substances not intended for household use. https://www.cpsc.gov/s3fs-public/PPPA-Updated-Guidance-on-Substances-Not-Intended-for-Household-Use.pdf. Accessed 21 Aug 2025.
22. Lander L, Howsare J, Byrne M. The impact of substance use disorders on families and children: from theory to practice. Soc Work Public Health. 2013;28(3-4):194–205. https://doi.org/10.1080/19371918.2013.759005.
23. Hogue A, Becker SJ, Wenzel K, et al. Family involvement in treatment and recovery for substance use disorders among transition-age youth: research bedrocks and opportunities. J Subst Abuse Treat. 2021;129:108402. https://doi.org/10.1016/j.jsat.2021.108402.
24. Hogue A, Brykman K, Guilamo-Ramos V, et al. Family-focused universal substance use prevention in primary care: advancing a pragmatic national healthcare agenda. Prev Sci. 2024;25(2):307–17. https://doi.org/10.1007/s11121-023-01584-4.
25. Gaither JR, McCollum S, Bechtel K, Leventhal JM, Mintz S. The circumstances surrounding fatal pediatric opioid poisonings, 2004–2020. Pediatrics. 2024;154(Suppl 3). https://doi.org/10.1542/peds.2024-067043N.
26. Bountress K, Chassin L. Risk for behavior problems in children of parents with substance use disorders. Am J Orthopsychiatry. 2015;85(3):275–86. https://doi.org/10.1037/ort0000063.
27. Winstanley EL, Stover AN. The impact of the opioid epidemic on children and adolescents. Clin Ther. 2019;41(9):1655–62. https://doi.org/10.1016/j.clinthera.2019.06.003.
28. Marsh JC, Smith BD. Integrated substance abuse and child welfare services for women: a progress review. Child Youth Serv Rev. 2011;33(3):466–72. https://doi.org/10.1016/j.childyouth.2010.06.017.
29. Adams ZM, Ginapp CM, Price CR, et al. "A good mother": impact of motherhood identity on women's substance use and engagement in treatment across the lifespan. J Subst Abuse Treat. 2021;130:108474. https://doi.org/10.1016/j.jsat.2021.108474.
30. Szilagyi MA, Rosen DS, Rubin D, et al. Health care issues for children and adolescents in foster care and kinship care. Pediatrics. 2015;136(4):e1142–66. https://doi.org/10.1542/peds.2015-2656.
31. Szilagyi M. The pediatric role in the care of children in foster and kinship care. Pediatr Rev. 2012;33(11):496–507.; quiz 508. https://doi.org/10.1542/pir.33-11-496.
32. Yale School of Medicine/Child Study Center. Family-Based Recovery Services. https://medicine.yale.edu/childstudy/education-and-training/professional-development/family-based-recovery-services/. Accessed 15 Sept 2022.
33. Suchman NE, DeCoste CL, McMahon TJ, Dalton R, Mayes LC, Borelli J. Mothering from the inside out: results of a second randomized clinical trial testing a mentalization-based intervention for mothers in addiction treatment. Dev Psychopathol. 2017;29(2):617–36. https://doi.org/10.1017/S0954579417000220.
34. Suchman N, Pajulo M, Decoste C, Mayes L. Parenting interventions for drug-dependent mothers and their young children: the case for an attachment-based approach. Fam Relat. 2006;55(2):211–26. https://doi.org/10.1111/j.1741-3729.2006.00371.x.
35. Substance Abuse and Mental Health Services Administration. Counselor's family education manual. https://library.samhsa.gov/sites/default/files/sma13-4153.pdf. Accessed 21 Aug 2025.
36. Yale Program in Addiction Medicine. Central Medical Unit, APT Foundation. https://medicine.yale.edu/internal-medicine/genmed/addictionmedicine/clinical/cmu/. Accessed 21 Aug 2025.
37. APT Foundation. Substance use treatment. https://aptfoundation.org/#. Accessed 21 Aug 2025.
38. Meta House. Ending the generational cycle of addiction by healing women and strengthening families. https://www.milwaukeemhtf.org/wp-content/uploads/2023/01/MHTF-Meta-House-Presentation-01-2023.pdf. Accessed 21 Aug 2025.
39. University of Pennsylvania. The Center for High Impact Philanthropy. Meta House. https://www.impact.upenn.edu/high-impact-giving-guide-2019/meta-house/. Accessed 21 Aug 2025.
40. Grossman MR, Berkwitt AK, Osborn RR, et al. An initiative to improve the quality of care of infants with neonatal abstinence syndrome. Pediatrics. 2017;139(6). https://doi.org/10.1542/peds.2016-3360.

References

41. Grossman MR, Lipshaw MJ, Osborn RR, Berkwitt AK. A novel approach to assessing infants with neonatal abstinence syndrome. Hosp Pediatr. 2018;8(1):1–6. https://doi.org/10.1542/hpeds.2017-0128.
42. Young LW, Ounpraseuth ST, Merhar SL, et al. Eat, sleep, console approach or usual care for neonatal opioid withdrawal. N Engl J Med. 2023;388(25):2326–37. https://doi.org/10.1056/NEJMoa2214470.

8

What Can We Learn from Other Countries, Past Eras?

The United States stands alone among developed nations in both healthcare spending and the devastating scope of its opioid epidemic. Despite investing more in healthcare than any other developed country in the world, America has significantly poorer health outcomes across a variety of conditions. These disparities are particularly stark for opioid misuse, addiction, and overdose. Prior to the 1990s, the United States had conservative opioid prescribing practices, similar to those of other nations, but shifts in approaches to pain management, drug potency, and aggressive pharmaceutical marketing fundamentally reshaped standards of care for opioid use in the United States. This chapter explores how these changes contributed to global disparities in opioid consumption and adverse effects. Germany, Japan, and several Nordic countries have implemented safer and more effective approaches to opioid prescribing, addiction treatment, and social services. Despite having aging populations with high pain management needs, these countries have avoided the public health catastrophe seen in the United States through tighter regulatory controls, universal healthcare coverage for nonopioid treatments, and integrated primary care models for addiction treatment. Understanding these differences in approaches, particularly as they relate to family-centered care, offers valuable lessons for gaining control of the crisis in the United States.

8.1 Global Perspectives: Learning from International Approaches to Opioid Safety

While previous chapters have outlined systemic reforms needed within the United States to protect families from opioids, this chapter examines how other nations have approached opioid safety. Despite comparable levels of pain management needs and healthcare complexities, many developed nations have avoided the public health devastation seen in the United States from opioid misuse, addiction, and mortality. These international models offer concrete examples of how the family-centered, integrated approaches advocated for in Chap. 7 can be successfully implemented on a national scale, particularly regarding opioid prescribing practices, healthcare integration, and family support.

The stark contrast in drug overdose mortality between the United States and other developed nations is staggering. Recent data from the Commonwealth Fund reveals that Americans are dying from drug overdoses at dramatically higher rates than other high-income countries [1, 2]. In 2021, according to the Commonwealth Fund, the United States had the highest overdose morality rate in the world at approximately 320 per million residents, followed by Scotland at 267 and Canada at 171 per million. All other countries had rates below 100 per million, with Norway at approximately 60 deaths per million, Germany at 19, and France at 7 [1]. When considering these statistics, it is important to note that methodologies for classifying and reporting deaths vary by country. Even after accounting for these differences, however, the disparities in the data suggest that healthcare delivery systems, prescribing practices, drug policies, and regulatory frameworks play a decisive role in mitigating overdose risks [3].

8.2 The Widening Gap: How the Opioid Crisis Exacerbates America's Health Disparities

America spends more on healthcare than any other developed nation but has poorer outcomes—particularly for women and children [2, 4–6]. This is a longstanding problem, and until recently, the major contributors were higher mortality rates among infants—largely attributable to poor prenatal care for birthing mothers—and poor nutrition due to poverty [7]. The opioid crisis has served to widen these gaps among women and children as well as the general population [8–12].

In 2024, researchers at Virginia Commonwealth University published a study showing that easier access to opioids and guns has led to greater disparities in the health of children [13]. The authors showed that relative to 16 other high-income countries, the United States has higher mortality rates for infants, children, and adolescents. Between 1999 and 2019, there were over 400,000 excess deaths among children aged 0–19 years, averaging approximately 20,000 deaths per year. More than half of these deaths were among infants, the group that has traditionally had the highest mortality rates. Excess deaths among teenagers 15–19 years of age accounted for more than 25% of excess deaths. The opioid crisis has also reduced life expectancy [14], further widening health disparities between the United States and much of the developed world, underscoring the urgent need for systemic changes in opioid prevention and substance use treatment in this country.

8.3 Controlled Prescribing Practices

While most countries have been able to avoid the devastating epidemic experienced in America from opioids, Germany offers perhaps the most compelling case study—and the most instructive. Germany is the most populous country in the European

8.3 Controlled Prescribing Practices

Union and has the largest economy. Germany, despite similar overall levels of opioid use as the United States, has avoided the widespread rates of addiction and mortality seen in America [3], largely through systems that control opioid prescribing and early intervention for those who show signs of a substance use disorder [1].

As reported by German researchers in a 2019 study, drug overdose deaths are a tiny fraction of what they are in the United States [15]. After examining data from inpatient and outpatient treatment facilities in Germany and the country's opioid substitution registry, the researchers found that between 2000 and 2016, the rate of opioid addiction did not increase dramatically, and the number of people addicted in 2016 was only 0.2% (or 166,300) of Germany's population. During the same timeframe in the United States, the prevalence of opioid addiction rose by over 300%.

For opioid fatalities, Germany's overdose mortality rate saw little change from 2007 to 2016 [15]. In contrast, between 2001 and 2016 in the United States, opioid fatalities increased 345% [16].

This stark difference stems largely from how Germany approaches opioid prescribing and pain management. As explained by Dr. Peter Raiser, director of the German Center for Addiction Issues: "Among the most important reasons we do not face a similar opioid crisis [in Germany] seems to be a more responsible and restrained practice of prescription" [15]. According to Dr. Raiser, in Germany, opioids have never been seen as the first treatment option for either acute or chronic pain. For physicians who do want to prescribe opioids, they must first get permission to do so and screen patients to ensure that the risk of addiction is low. Opioids are seen as an option only after all others have been considered. "Here in Germany, they prescribe opiates if all the other drugs don't work," states Dr. Dieter Naber of the University of Hamburg.

Germany has managed to allow access to opioids for legitimate pain management while maintaining rational regulatory oversight of the drugs and lower prescribing rates than the United States. This balanced approach recognizes the importance of opioids for pain management while adhering to safeguards that mitigate the risk of misuse.

Another key difference that helps explain why Germany has avoided the problems seen in America lies in where opioids are used—largely within institutional settings rather than outpatient facilities. Germany's high per capita opioid consumption rate is driven primarily by hospital use (e.g., fentanyl for inpatient surgery). Thus, there is far less medically unsupervised use of opioids in Germany, which means that fewer of the drugs accumulate in homes and medicine cabinets, where they can be accessed by anyone—including children and adolescents.

The complex relationship between opioid prescribing and overdose deaths deserves particular attention. While America's crisis began with prescription opioids, international data reveal that the volume of opioids prescribed is not the sole determinant of overdose mortality. Several countries have been able to maintain high rates of opioid consumption without incurring epidemic-level consequences. The key difference appears to be how opioids are integrated into healthcare systems that offer more comprehensive levels of care, prescribe according to evidence-based protocols, and have the infrastructure in place to provide more robust safety nets, particularly for addiction treatment.

Building on the lessons from Germany, additional insights can be gained from how Nordic countries have avoided an opioid crisis by closely monitoring opioid prescribing. Like Germany, most Nordic countries have implemented multiple measures that have kept rates of opioid addiction and fatalities far lower than those seen in the United States. In general, Nordic countries have a tradition of more restrictive regulatory frameworks for opioid prescribing that emphasize appropriate use for severe pain while encouraging opioid alternatives, when possible, such as physical and behavioral therapies. As in Germany, these alternatives are covered by universal healthcare models. These countries also limit the quantity of opioids that are dispensed at one time. All five Nordic countries (Denmark, Finland, Iceland, Norway, and Sweden) have nationwide prescription drug monitoring programs that track all dispensed medications and allow for real-time surveillance of prescriptions. Because these systems link to other national data repositories, including electronic medical records, they enable comprehensive monitoring of drug safety and effectiveness [17].

Japan's approach to pain management also contrasts sharply with America's approach, despite having an aging population and high healthcare utilization. Per capita use of six of the most commonly prescribed opioids—including buprenorphine, morphine, methadone, and fentanyl—was 26 times higher in the United States compared to Japan [18]. In part, this dates back to changes in legislation from the early nineteenth century enacted to control the use of opioids, which are still highly regulated. Under Japan's national healthcare system, strict procedures must be followed before insurance will cover the use of opioids. For example, oxycodone will only be covered if used to treat cancer pain; it cannot be prescribed for acute or chronic noncancer pain. In contrast, tramadol combined with acetaminophen is only covered if used for noncancer pain and tooth extraction, while codeine, morphine, and fentanyl can be prescribed for both cancer and noncancer pain [18].

8.4 Structure of Healthcare Systems and Universal Insurance Coverage

Germany has a universal healthcare system, which requires physicians to be more judicious in how opioids are prescribed. Before starting opioids, doctors must first try other treatments, including nonpharmaceutical approaches that are covered by insurance. In contrast, in the United States, insurance companies are unlikely to pay for anything other than a prescription to treat chronic pain. According to Professor Judith Feinberg of West Virginia University, "Most insurance, especially for poor people, won't pay for anything but a pill." Dr. Feinberg, a prominent figure in the field of opioids research and its impact on low-income communities, particularly in her state of West Virginia, elaborates: "Say you have a patient that's 45 years old. They have lower back pain, you examine them, they have a muscle spasm. Really the best thing is physical therapy, but no one will pay for that. So, doctors get ready to pull out the prescription pad" [19].

In Japan, before a physician can prescribe opioids for chronic noncancer pain, the doctor must have completed lengthy e-training modules specific to each type of opioid to be prescribed. Additionally, both the physician and patient must sign a contractual agreement before opioid treatment begins [18]. Perhaps most importantly, nonopioid analgesics must be tried first.

8.5 Addiction Treatment Integration and Provider Training

In addition to prescribing controls and access to affordable alternative treatments, Germany also has more harm reduction measures in place to help people—all of which have helped to keep addiction rates and fatalities low in the country. Germany's success with its multipronged approach illustrates that addiction is "a more complex problem" than the current American response has acknowledged, according to Dr. Raiser [20].

Germany manages this complexity in its approach to addiction treatment for patients who do develop a substance use disorder [21]. With its emphasis on primary care and the low cost of receiving medical care, patients are more likely to keep their doctor's appointments. Warning signs of addiction are thus more likely to be noticed early by doctors, allowing them to get patients into treatment, which is also covered by universal insurance. Like with many European countries, the approach to addiction treatment is comprehensive, accessible, and focused on prevention and early intervention [21, 22].

Primary care doctors play a central role in this system of care. For individuals experiencing substance use disorders, family doctors are often the first point of contact. Many of the general practitioners who help patients gain access to treatment have themselves received specific training in addiction medicine. In contrast, primary care doctors in the United States receive little training in addiction medicine, which significantly limits their ability to recognize and treat substance use disorders. Given how prevalent substance use disorders are in the United States, this is a major barrier to care for families in this country, where primary care and addiction medicine remain fragmented [23].

The importance of training physicians in the United States to recognize and screen for substance use disorders becomes clearer when you consider the scope of the problem of substance use in the United States. It is currently estimated that one-third of adults seen in primary care in the United States suffer from a substance use disorder [24]. This is according to the Substance Abuse and Mental Health Services Administration (SAMHSA), an agency within the Department of Health and Human Services (HHS), which each year releases an annual survey designed to provide estimates of the prevalence of substance use and mental health disorders in the United States. According to the National Survey on Drug Use and Health (NSDUH), there were approximately 48.5 million Americans over the age of 12 who met the DSM-5 (*Diagnostic Statistical Manual*, fifth edition) criteria for past-year substance use disorder in 2023 [25]. These data show that nearly 17% of Americans 12 and over engaged in illicit drug use in the prior 12 months—all of which underscore the importance of integrating addiction medicine into primary care for adults, adolescents, and parents of small children [23, 26].

8.6 Cultural Factors

Beyond specific policies and programs, broader cultural and systemic factors significantly influence how countries respond to potential opioid crises. Understanding these differences helps explain why similar levels of opioid prescribing have led to vastly different outcomes across nations [27].

Cultural differences in how pain is perceived and treated vary substantially across different societies. *Patients in the United States, where drugs are marketed directly to consumers (like any other commodity), have different expectations about what medicine should be able to do for them.* According to Dr. Feinberg, "Other countries deal with pain in healthier ways" [19].

In the United States, pharmaceutical marketing directly to consumers—which is prohibited in most other developed nations—has fundamentally shaped patient expectations about pain management. Americans are uniquely exposed to advertising that suggests there should be a pharmaceutical solution for every type of discomfort.

The structure of the American healthcare system, with its fragmented coverage and focus on fee-for-service care, creates perverse incentives that favor quick solutions like prescriptions over comprehensive pain management approaches. The US practice of tying health insurance to employment means that severely addicted people often lose access to treatment at precisely the time they need it most.

Cultural attitudes toward pain itself differ significantly across societies. As pain researcher Mark Sullivan has noted, Americans tend to view pain as something that should be eliminated entirely, while other cultures view some level of pain as a normal part of life that can be managed rather than eradicated [28]. In Japan, for example, there are societal mores that prevent patients from complaining about pain, and the use of opioids for treating chronic noncancer pain is not culturally sanctioned [18]. In fact, it is frowned upon.

8.7 Historical Perspectives: America's Changing Approach

It is also insightful to review the history of opioids in this country and how America's departure from its own conservative opioid practices contributed to the current epidemic. As noted in Chap. 1, US prescribing practices and regulations have evolved substantially over time. Prior to the 1990s, opioid prescribing in the United States was much more conservative, with strong regulatory controls limiting their use primarily to cancer and end-of-life care [29]. The medical community generally viewed opioids as inappropriate for chronic noncancer pain due to concerns about addiction [30].

This changed dramatically in the mid-1990s with the introduction of the "Pain as the 5th Vital Sign" initiative and the aggressive marketing by pharmaceutical companies like Purdue Pharma [31]. The American Pain Society's campaign to improve pain treatment, while well-intentioned, created pressure on physicians to prescribe more opioids [32].

The pharmaceutical industry's influence on medical education, research, and clinical guidelines further accelerated the shift toward liberal opioid prescribing [31, 33–36]. Unlike in countries with more centralized healthcare systems, the United States lacked robust mechanisms to counterbalance industry marketing with objective prescribing guidance.

Past regulatory successes in the United States demonstrate that effective regulation of potentially harmful medications is possible [37]. However, the political will to implement similar controls for opioids was undermined by industry influence and shifting cultural attitudes toward pain management.

8.8   Lessons from Other Countries and the Past

Drawing from international comparisons and historical lessons, several key principles emerge that could guide more effective approaches to the opioid crisis in the United States.

Regulated prescribing practices must be paired with accessible alternatives. Germany's success stems not just from restricting opioid access but from ensuring that patients have access to pain management approaches that are covered by insurance. As we have seen in the United States, attempts to limit opioid prescribing without simultaneously expanding access and coverage for nonopioid therapies fail because patients either turn to the misuse of prescription or illicit substances or are left without adequate pain management [38–40]. These nonopioid alternatives include mental health interventions, such as cognitive-behavioral therapy and physical therapy.

Healthcare systems in the United States must better integrate addiction treatment into primary care. The stark contrast between Germany's early intervention approach and America's fragmented specialty care model underscores the benefits of routine care with doctors who are familiar with a patient's history. This familiarity allows for early intervention when the warning signs of addiction appear. Treatment in these early stages is likely to be more effective clinically and cost less.

In Germany, primary care doctors receive specific training in addiction medicine and serve as the first point of contact for individuals suffering from substance use disorders. This integrated approach allows for early detection and intervention and the chance to halt the progression to a severe disorder that would otherwise require intensive and costly treatment. Given the prevalence of substance use disorders in the United States, primary care physicians need better training in addiction medicine as well as the time and resources to address substance use alongside other health concerns.

The international and historical evidence provides concrete examples of how the systemic reforms advocated for in Chap. 7 can be successfully implemented on a national scale. Specifically, reforms are needed in the following areas:

1. Adoption of balanced regulatory frameworks that recognize the legitimate use of opioids for pain while also recognizing that appropriate safeguards are needed in how and when the drugs are prescribed and adverse effects monitored
2. Expansion of insurance coverage for comprehensive pain management approaches that include physical therapy, psychological interventions, and complementary alternative modalities that are currently underutilized because of financial barriers and incentives
3. Implementation of standardized pain assessment protocols and evidence-based prescribing guidelines that focus on functional improvement rather than eliminating pain entirely
4. Changes in policy that limit direct-to-consumer marketing of prescription drugs, which often establish unrealistic expectations of what medications can do, especially regarding pain relief

These approaches have proven successful in countries that have vastly different cultural and political contexts.

But it is important to note that there is one crucial area where all nations are falling short: globally, few examples exist of the family-centered models that I have advocated for in this book. The opioid crisis represents an opportunity for American to position itself as a leader with innovative models that address the intergenerational impact of substance use. Specifically, the United States has the opportunity to develop integrated systems that, at their core, recognize the extent to which substance use affects entire families.

As we turn our attention in the next chapter to opioid settlement funds, we face a historic opportunity to reshape America's approach to the opioid crisis. The billions of dollars now flowing to states and communities from settlements with pharmaceutical companies represent perhaps our best chance to implement these lessons from abroad—creating integrated healthcare approaches, expanding access to nonopioid treatments, and developing family-centered models of care that prioritize child safety alongside adult recovery.

References

1. The Commonwealth Fund. Too many lives lost: comparing overdose mortality rates and policy solutions across high-income countries. https://www.commonwealthfund.org/blog/2022/too-many-lives-lost-comparing-overdose-mortality-rates-policy-solutions. Accessed 18 Jan 2025.
2. Blumenthal D, Gumas E, Shah A. The failing U.S. health system. N Engl J Med. 2024;391(17):1566–8. https://doi.org/10.1056/NEJMp2410855.
3. Humphreys K. What the US can learn from other countries to combat the opioid crisis. https://www.brookings.edu/articles/what-the-us-and-canada-can-learn-from-other-countries-to-

combat-the-opioid-crisis/#:~:text=Key%20lessons%20include%20that%20flooding,are%20 prescribed%20matter%2C%20among%20others. Accessed 1 Mar 2025.
4. The Commonwealth Fund. Mirror, mirror 2024: a portrait of the failing U.S. health system. Comparing performance in 10 nations. https://www.commonwealthfund.org/publications/fund-reports/2024/sep/mirror-mirror-2024. Accessed 22 Aug 2025.
5. The Commonwealth Fund. Healthcare for women: how the U.S. compares internationally. https://www.commonwealthfund.org/publications/issue-briefs/2024/aug/health-care-women-how-us-compares-internationally. Accessed 22 Aug 2025.
6. Forrest CB, Koenigsberg LJ, Eddy Harvey F, Maltenfort MG, Halfon N. Trends in US children's mortality, chronic conditions, obesity, functional status, and symptoms. JAMA. 2025;334(6):509–16. https://doi.org/10.1001/jama.2025.9855.
7. Chehab RF, Croen LA, Laraia BA, et al. Food insecurity in pregnancy, receipt of food assistance, and perinatal complications. JAMA Netw Open. 2025;8(1):e2455955. https://doi.org/10.1001/jamanetworkopen.2024.55955.
8. Gaither JR, Shabanova V, Leventhal JM. US national trends in pediatric deaths from prescription and illicit opioids, 1999–2016. JAMA Netw Open. 2018;1(8):e186558. https://doi.org/10.1001/jamanetworkopen.2018.6558.
9. Gaither JR, McCollum S, Bechtel K, Leventhal JM, Mintz S. The circumstances surrounding fatal pediatric opioid poisonings, 2004–2020. Pediatrics. 2024;154(Suppl 3). https://doi.org/10.1542/peds.2024-067043N.
10. Gaither JR. National trends in pediatric deaths from fentanyl, 1999–2021. JAMA Pediatr. 2023. https://doi.org/10.1001/jamapediatrics.2023.0793.
11. Goldstick JE, Cunningham RM, Carter PM. Current causes of death in children and adolescents in the United States. N Engl J Med. 2022;386(20):1955–6. https://doi.org/10.1056/NEJMc2201761.
12. Bond GR, Woodward RW, Ho M. The growing impact of pediatric pharmaceutical poisoning. J Pediatr. 2012;160(2):265–270.e1. https://doi.org/10.1016/j.jpeds.2011.07.042.
13. Woolf SH, Chapman DA. Excess US deaths attributable to high all-cause mortality rates among youths aged 0 to 19 years. JAMA Pediatr. 2024;178(9):942–4. https://doi.org/10.1001/jamapediatrics.2024.1869.
14. Association of American Medical Colleges. Narrowing the gap: the burden of alcohol, drugs, and firearms on U.S. life expectancy. https://www.aamc.org/advocacy-policy/publication/narrowing-gap-burden-alcohol-drugs-and-firearms-us-life-expectancy. Accessed 22 Aug 2025.
15. Addiction Center. The opioid epidemic in Germany. https://www.addictioncenter.com/news/2020/02/opioid-addiction-germany-united-states/. Accessed 18 Jan 2025.
16. Gomes T, Tadrous M, Mamdani MM, Paterson JM, Juurlink DN. The burden of opioid-related mortality in the United States. JAMA Netw Open. 2018;1(2):e180217. https://doi.org/10.1001/jamanetworkopen.2018.0217.
17. Wettermark B, Zoega H, Furu K, et al. The Nordic prescription databases as a resource for pharmacoepidemiological research—a literature review. Pharmacoepidemiol Drug Saf. 2013;22(7):691–9. https://doi.org/10.1002/pds.3457.
18. Onishi E, Kobayashi T, Dexter E, Marino M, Maeno T, Deyo RA. Comparison of opioid prescribing patterns in the United States and Japan: primary care physicians' attitudes and perceptions. J Am Board Fam Med. 2017;30(2):248–54. https://doi.org/10.3122/jabfm.2017.02.160299.
19. BBC News. Why opioids are such an American problem. https://www.bbc.com/news/world-us-canada-41701718. Accessed 1 Mar 2025.
20. KIPU Health. Germany's approach to addiction. https://www.kipuhealth.com/resources/germanys-approach-to-addiction/. Accessed 22 Aug 2025.
21. Drug Policy Facts. Substance use treatment in Germany. https://www.drugpolicyfacts.org/node/4052. Accessed 22 Aug 2025.
22. European Union Drugs Agency. Germany, country drug report 2019. https://www.euda.europa.eu/publications/country-drug-reports/2019/germany_en. Accessed 22 Aug 2019.

23. Hogue A, Brykman K, Guilamo-Ramos V, et al. Family-focused universal substance use prevention in primary care: advancing a pragmatic national healthcare agenda. Prev Sci. 2024;25(2):307–17. https://doi.org/10.1007/s11121-023-01584-4.
24. Substance Abuse and Mental Health Services Administration. National survey on drug use and health. https://www.samhsa.gov/data/data-we-collect/nsduh-national-survey-drug-use-and-health/national-releases/older. Accessed 18 Jan 2025.
25. Substance Abuse and Mental Health Services Administration. Key substance use and mental health indicators in the United States: results from the 2023 national survey on drug use and health. https://www.samhsa.gov/data/sites/default/files/reports/rpt47095/National%20Report/National%20Report/2023-nsduh-annual-national.htm. Accessed 22 Aug 2025.
26. Hogue A, Becker SJ, Wenzel K, et al. Family involvement in treatment and recovery for substance use disorders among transition-age youth: research bedrocks and opportunities. J Subst Abus Treat. 2021;129:108402. https://doi.org/10.1016/j.jsat.2021.108402.
27. Duff JH, Library of Congress. Congressional Research Service. Consumption of prescription opioids for pain : a comparison of opioid use in the United States and other countries. Library of Congress public edition, ed. Report / Congressional Research Service R46805. Congressional Research Service; 2021.
28. Sullivan M. Four myths that helped cause the opioid epidemic. https://markdsullivan.org/four-myths-that-helped-cause-the-opioid-epidemic/. Accessed 22 Aug.
29. Fischer B, Rehm J. Revisiting the 'paradigm shift' in opioid use: developments and implications 10 years later. Drug Alcohol Rev. 2018;37(Suppl 1):S199–202. https://doi.org/10.1111/dar.12539.
30. Von Korff M, Kolodny A, Deyo RA, Chou R. Long-term opioid therapy reconsidered. Ann Intern Med. 2011;155(5):325–8. https://doi.org/10.7326/0003-4819-155-5-201109060-00011.
31. Van Zee A. The promotion and marketing of oxycontin: commercial triumph, public health tragedy. Am J Public Health. 2009;99(2):221–7. https://doi.org/10.2105/AJPH.2007.131714.
32. Humble W. The 5th vital sign: the painkiller epidemic part I of V. 2014. https://directorsblog.health.azdhs.gov/the-5th-vital-sign-the-painkiller-epidemic-part-i-of-v/. Accessed 14 June 2024.
33. Spithoff S, Leece P, Sullivan F, Persaud N, Belesiotis P, Steiner L. Drivers of the opioid crisis: an appraisal of financial conflicts of interest in clinical practice guideline panels at the peak of opioid prescribing. PLoS One. 2020;15(1):e0227045. https://doi.org/10.1371/journal.pone.0227045.
34. Erdek MA. What clinicians and health professions students should learn about how pharmaceutical marketing influences opioid prescribing and patient outcomes. AMA J Ethics. 2020;22(1):E681–6. https://doi.org/10.1001/amajethics.2020.681.
35. Hadland SE, Cerda M, Li Y, Krieger MS, Marshall BDL. Association of pharmaceutical industry marketing of opioid products to physicians with subsequent opioid prescribing. JAMA Intern Med. 2018;178(6):861–3. https://doi.org/10.1001/jamainternmed.2018.1999.
36. Kesselheim AS, Avorn J, Sarpatwari A. The high cost of prescription drugs in the United States: origins and prospects for reform. JAMA. 2016;316(8):858–71. https://doi.org/10.1001/jama.2016.11237.
37. Carpenter DP, ebrary Inc. Reputation and power organizational image and pharmaceutical regulation at the FDA. Princeton University Press; 2010:xx, 802 p. https://yale.idm.oclc.org/login?URL=http://site.ebrary.com/lib/yale/Doc?id=10394772.
38. Gaither JR, Goulet JL, Becker WC, et al. Guideline-concordant management of opioid therapy among human immunodeficiency virus (HIV)-infected and uninfected veterans. J Pain. 2014;15(11):1130–40. https://doi.org/10.1016/j.jpain.2014.08.004.
39. Gaither JR, Goulet JL, Becker WC, et al. The effect of substance use disorders on the association between guideline-concordant long-term opioid therapy and all-cause mortality. J Addict Med. 2016;10(6):418–28. https://doi.org/10.1097/ADM.0000000000000255.
40. Gaither JR, Goulet JL, Becker WC, et al. The association between receipt of guideline-concordant long-term opioid therapy and all-cause mortality. J Gen Intern Med. 2016;31(5):492–501. https://doi.org/10.1007/s11606-015-3571-4.

Opioid Settlement Funds: An Opportunity for States to Prioritize Children

9

This chapter explores how the national opioid settlement funds represent an unprecedented opportunity for the United States to prioritize children as it attempts to repair the damage caused by opioids to families and communities across the nation. As a result of hundreds of lawsuits brought on behalf of more than 3000 local and state entities, numerous companies involved in the manufacture, sale, distribution, or marketing of opioids are expected to pay out approximately $50 billion over the next two decades. Advisory committees have been established in most states to guide the allocation of these funds. While most committees include representation from adults with substance use disorders, they often fail to include families who have lost children to opioid poisonings. This oversight reflects a broader societal trend in prioritizing adult needs over child safety. Drawing on research showing that pediatric opioid poisonings continue unabated even as adult overdose rates may be stabilizing, I propose age-specific and evidence-based interventions that will ensure that funds are allocated to address the needs of children.

9.1 National Opioid Litigation and Settlements

The opioid settlement funds present a once-in-a-generation opportunity to address the lack of protections afforded to children over the past three decades of the opioid crisis. With more than $50 billion expected to flow to state and local governments over the next two decades, the scale of the resources available is unprecedented.

The settlement stems from hundreds of ongoing lawsuits between state, local, and tribal governments and the pharmaceutical industry. The largest settlement to date is between Johnson & Johnson (J&J), AmerisourceBergen, Cardinal Health, and McKesson and 46 states, which in July 2021 received $26 billion in settlement funds. In addition to funds awarded through what is referred to as the "National Settlement," J&J and three opioid distributors have agreed to pay $590 million to Native American tribes and tribal health organizations (Native Americans have experienced some of the highest overdose rates in the country) [1, 2].

Settlements have also been reached with several pharmacies and retailers—including CVS, Walgreens, and Walmart—who have agreed to pay $13.8 billion to settle lawsuits with state, local, and tribal governments.

Also included in the $50 billion total is the roughly $8 billion expected from a controversial settlement between state and local governments as well as individual plaintiffs and Purdue Pharma, the makers of OxyContin, which as of this writing (August 2025) is tied up in US bankruptcy court. In 2019, the Sackler family, which owns Purdue, attempted to shield themselves from lawsuits by letting the company go bankrupt. As part of the bankruptcy negotiations, the company agreed to pay $6 billion to settle existing lawsuits but sought immunity from further litigation. Prior to filing for bankruptcy, however, the family moved approximately $11 billion in company profits into personal family accounts. This deal, which was approved by a federal US bankruptcy judge in 2021, was overturned in a 5–4 decision by the Supreme Court in July 2024 [3]. A new deal worth $7.4 billion, which includes 900 million from Purdue's assets, was announced in January 2025 and approved by the bankruptcy court in June. A confirmation hearing is set for November 2025. If approved, $850 million of the $7.5 billion is earmarked to directly compensate individuals who either lost a family member to opioids or accrued substantial expenses related to addiction treatment or the birth of a child with NOWS [4]. Given that there are approximately 140,000 individual claimants, the payouts will be small for most individuals, from a minimum of $3500 to a maximum in the range of $40,000 for a death [5].

9.2 The Framework: Distribution of Funds and Mechanisms for Oversight

The negotiated agreement between the pharmaceutical companies, including Johnson & Johnson, opioid distributors, and state attorneys generally stipulates that 70% of funds must be spent on "opioid remediation efforts" that (1) address the misuse and abuse of opioids, (2) treat or mitigate opioid disorders, or (3) mitigate the effects of the opioid epidemic, including as it relates to those who were injured by opioids.

The settlement includes specific mechanisms for ensuring that the funds are spent appropriately and to avoid a repeat of what occurred with the 1998 Tobacco Master Settlement Agreement between state governments and the four largest tobacco companies ("Big Tobacco"). Less than 3% of the $35 billion received by states was spent on smoking prevention and cessation programs [6]. For the opioid settlement, each of the 46 states participating is required to establish an Opioid Settlement Remediation Advisory Committee. The role of these committees is to provide input and offer recommendations on how the funds should be spent. According to the settlement agreement, to ensure a balance of power, committees must have equal representation at both the state and local levels, include a process for receiving input from the public, and establish processes through which state agencies consider public recommendations.

The composition of these advisory committees varies by state, but common patterns have emerged in who has been given a voice in how the funds are spent. Most states require representation from elected officials, providers who treat substance use, and members of the recovery community. Seven states (Colorado, Maine, Massachusetts, Montana, Oregon, Texas, and Virginia) take community involvement a step further by requiring committees to include those with "lived experience," an individual with a past or current opioid use disorder or an affected family member [7, 8]. Several states have gone beyond these requirements, actively soliciting public engagement by asking for feedback from communities on how the funds should be spent [9, 10]. According to an analysis by the Kaiser Family Foundation, Shatterproof (a non-profit advocating for the use of the settlement funds to treat opioid addiction), and Johns Hopkins Bloomberg School of Public Health, only 7% of seats nationwide are currently filled by members of the public citing lived experience [8, 11].

9.3 Funding Priorities: Five Guiding Principles and Nine Core Strategies

Although state and local governments ultimately control how their share of the opioid settlement funds will be spent, national guidelines have been established to direct the spending and allocation of the funds [12]. These guiding principles were established by faculty and staff at Johns Hopkins Bloomberg School of Public Health as part of the Bloomberg Overdose Prevention Initiative and in collaboration with organizations across the field of substance use. According to the website and national dashboard set up by Johns Hopkins, governments are encouraged to be "good stewards of restitution dollars" and adopt five principles when making funding decisions [12]:

1. Spend the money to save lives
   - Establish a dedicated fund in which to put the dollars
   - Use the dollars to supplement rather than supplant existing funding
   - Don't spend all the money at once
2. Use evidence to guide spending
3. Invest in primary prevention efforts targeted at youth
4. Focus on racial equity
5. Develop a fair and transparent process for deciding where to spend the funding

In addition to these guiding principles, the national settlement outlines nine core opioid abatement strategies/populations that governments are encouraged to prioritize [13]:

1. Naloxone
2. Prevention programs
3. Pregnant and postpartum women

4. NAS/NOWS treatment
5. Warm handoff and recovery services
6. Treatment for incarcerated population
7. Mothers with opioid use disorder
8. Expanding syringe service programs
9. Data collection and research

As required by the settlement, nearly all of the states have published guidelines on how they will allocate the funds, and each state has established unique structures and processes for identifying spending priorities, allocating funds across state and local entities, and ensuring transparency, accountability, and oversight.

9.4 Vulnerable Populations

Although the national guidelines encourage states to prioritize women and children affected by maternal OUD, only $8.4 million has been committed to caring for infants with NOWS. To date, less than 0.5% of these funds have actually been spent on this issue. The stigmatization of pregnant mothers with OUD likely plays a key role here. Women who use drugs, whether illicit or prescribed by a physician, are a highly stigmatized group. In my interviews of mothers with OUD, nearly every woman I spoke with described feeling judged by family and community members, including healthcare providers. One woman stated that she felt "branded" due to her history of substance use. This was a sentiment echoed by another mother who stated, "I guess because I have a past, and I've made bad choices, and because I'm on methadone, I [carry] a scarlet letter."

9.5 Promising Approaches: The Wisconsin Case Study

Wisconsin's community engagement model illustrates both the potential and the limitations of current initiatives and resource allocation [10]. The state, which is expected to receive $400 million from four separate settlements, held 12 regional online listening sessions prior to finalizing its plans for investing the opioid settlement funds. In total, nearly 600 people who were living with an opioid use disorder (or who had friends or family who were affected by the disorder), along with healthcare providers in the fields of opioid prevention, treatment, and recovery, participated in these virtual events. Nearly 900 additional comments were submitted through an online survey. According to the Wisconsin DHS website, several core themes for addressing the opioid epidemic emerged from the listening sessions:

- Addressing the root causes of the opioid crisis
- Improving access to mental health services
- Bolstering family stability

- Providing evidence-based substance use education to communities, especially in K-12 schools
- Enhancing harm reduction efforts related to naloxone access, fentanyl test strips, and safe injection sites
- Expanding accessibility of opioid use disorder treatment options
- Ensuring equity in the location and delivery of opioid use disorder treatment
- Supporting recovery by providing direct support to families affected by an opioid use disorder

One tangible outcome from this feedback was the Dose of Reality initiative, a collaboration between the Wisconsin Department of Health Services and the Department of Justice that aims to "change the conversation about the opioid epidemic in Wisconsin" by providing tools to prevent or reduce the risk of opioid use through "open and honest talks about the dangers of opioids and the way to save lives" [1, 8].

This initiative is notably comprehensive compared to other state efforts. It incorporates many of the core ideas covered in this book: improving public awareness through education and open discussions of basic safety measures such as safe storage and use of opioids, proper disposal of unused drugs, responding to an overdose, and getting help for an opioid use disorder. The program also broadens its reach beyond the public to address healthcare providers by including resources on best practices for pharmacists, prescribers, and "other professionals." Importantly, the initiative provides links to actual Wisconsin data and includes a marketing tool kit for disseminating information to the community through billboards, social media, and other channels.

Perhaps most notably, the Wisconsin initiative stands apart from similar state initiatives through its focus on encouraging individuals to initiate honest conversations with friends and family about opioids. The website provides practical tips on how to engage in such conversations as well as sample dialogue to help begin these discussions.

9.6 The Critical Gaps

Even Wisconsin's exemplary approach to educating the public about opioids, however, has persistent blind spots. The initiative falls short when it comes to women and children. While Wisconsin's focus on community dialogue represents a best practice that should be expanded nationally, it lacks the explicit inclusion of helping parents protect their families from opioids through conversations about opioid misuse, storage, disposal, and the risks to children. Indeed, the focus of all the conversational guidance pertains to helping someone who is misusing or abusing opioids. While the website does address the need to talk to adolescents about the dangers of substance use, it does not address the risks that opioids pose to young children and infants.

This gap in an otherwise comprehensive approach reflects broader patterns. Among all the initiatives I reviewed while researching this book, only a handful addressed children at all, and none comprehensively so. *More tellingly, while nearly all state committees included individuals with lived experience related to opioid use disorder, only a few included parents who had lost an adolescent to an overdose, and no committees included parents of young children who had died or had a close call because of an opioid poisoning.* This lack of representation reflects the low priority afforded to the impact of the opioid crisis on children in general and young children in particular.

Even the most comprehensive efforts fail to prioritize child safety. Wisconsin's approach, while exemplary in many ways, illustrates this pattern. The state has created several thoughtful initiatives aimed at adults with opioid use disorder, but these programs do not address children's safety.

From my research into the advisory committees, I know that slots have been allocated on the committees for people with "lived experience," specifically someone with personal experience with opioid addiction or recovery. These individuals should play a crucial role in guiding how the opioid settlement funds are allocated and will increase the chances that the programs and policies that are put in place actually serve the people that have been harmed by the crisis.

The absence of parents who have lost children to opioids from advisory committees is troubling. Those who understand the risks that opioids pose to children most intimately have no voice in how the settlement funds are allocated. Without parents and other child advocates at the table, opioids will likely remain a growing and persistent problem for the young in this country. Children's unique vulnerabilities to opioids will continue to be overlooked in favor of adult-centered interventions rather than family-centered solutions. This oversight occurs at the precise moment when we have both the resources and the knowledge to do better.

This exclusion of child advocates reflects a broader shift in how our society has come to understand and respond to substance use disorders—one that, while well-intentioned, may have inadvertently deprioritized child safety. This is the subject of a recent piece published by the American Enterprise Institute, a public policy think tank, entitled, "The U.S. Is Failing Substance Exposed Infants" [14], written by Dr. Sarah Font, an associate professor of sociology and public policy at Pennsylvania State University and a diverse team of researchers, child welfare advocates, and foundation leaders. In essence, the article asks whether, in an effort to improve the treatment of parents with substance use disorders, we are prioritizing their health and well-being over that of their children? The article states:

> Recent data on drug and alcohol use among pregnant women, pediatric poisonings, Narcan administrations to infants, and child fatalities all signal an unmitigated crisis. To date, however, the U.S. response has centered on parents and other adults experiencing addiction with inadequate attention to the needs of infants and young children in their care.

The article goes on to state:

> Individuals with substance use disorders may take many years to be "ready" for treatment, but there is no pause button on infants' development. Beyond the effects of prenatal substance

exposure itself, the effects of untreated substance use disorders on parenting are undeniable: Young children face increased risks of fatality, poisoning, injuries, physical and sexual abuse, and severe neglect, in addition to poor physical, cognitive, and emotional development.

In this article, Dr. Font and colleagues raise important ethical issues about how we balance our public health response to the opioid crisis. We do not face an either/or choice between supporting adults with substance use disorder and their children. The few family-centered models that have emerged in recent years demonstrate that it is possible to provide care that addresses both parental recovery and child safety simultaneously.

The disconnect between emerging adult-centered approaches and the persistent dangers to children that opioids pose is evident in recent reporting on the opioid crisis. Headlines across major newspapers are pointing to a potential turning point in the crisis based on modest decreases in adult overdose deaths over the past few years. On March 20, 2025, for example, the *Wall Street Journal* touted, "Drug Overdoses Decline as Use of Opioids Wanes." A headline a few months later tells a different story: On June 18, 2025, a headline from National Public Radio (NPR) read—"New Report: U.S. Drug Overdose Deaths Rise Again After Hopeful Decline." What this tells us is that it is too soon to celebrate. Whether opioid deaths are declining or not, *it is essential that Americans understand that opioids still claim around 100,000 lives every year.*

We must also consider whether the trends seen in adults apply to all age groups. There is no mention in these articles, or any of the dozens of others that I reviewed, of whether the trends seen in adults are also seen in children and adolescents. My research suggests that while there has been a slight decrease in opioid overdose deaths among older adolescents, deaths have not decreased among younger children. The opioid settlement funds provide an opportunity to correct this imbalance through targeted family-centered and age-specific interventions, but only if advocates have a seat at the table.

We must remain vigilant and continue to take concrete action. Settlement funds provide a unique opportunity to implement evidence-based protections for children. These must include:

- Age-specific prevention strategies that address the distinct risks faced by infants, young children, and adolescents from opioids
- Mandatory safety planning whenever opioids are prescribed to households with children
- Enhanced surveillance systems for tracking pediatric opioid exposures, hospitalizations, deaths, and near misses
- Expanded education for parents, caregivers, and healthcare providers about the specific dangers that opioids pose to children and how these vary by age
- Family-centered healthcare reforms that integrate addiction treatment with the care provided by pediatricians and child welfare providers

Settlement funds offer a critical opportunity to implement evidence-based protections that are specifically designed to protect our most vulnerable. We must ensure that the hard-earned lessons from this crisis translate into systems that will protect children not just from the current crisis, but from future drug epidemics.

References

1. Falkner R. Understanding opioid settlement spending plans across states: key components and approaches. https://nashp.org/understanding-opioid-settlement-spending-plans-across-states-key-components-and-approaches/. Accessed 1 Mar 2025.
2. Mann B. Supreme Court overturns opioid settlement with Purdue Pharma that shielded Sacklers. https://www.npr.org/sections/shots-health-news/2024/06/29/nx-s1-5021798/supreme-court-overturns-opioid-settlement-with-purdue-pharma-that-shielded-sacklerssupreme-court-overturns-sackler-settlement-delaying-funds-meant-for-communities-battling-opioids. Accessed 1 Mar 2025.
3. Supreme Court of the United States. Harrington, United States Trustee, Region 2 v. Purdue Pharma L. P. et al. Certiorari to the United States Court of Appeals for the Second Circuit. https://www.supremecourt.gov/opinions/23pdf/23-124_8nk0.pdf. Accessed 28 Aug 2025.
4. Purdue Pharma. Purdue Pharma L.P. receives court approval of disclosure statement filed in connection with its plan of reorganization. https://www.purduepharma.com/news/2025/06/20/purdue-pharma-l-p-receives-court-approval-of-disclosure-statement-filed-in-connection-with-its-plan-of-reorganization/. Accessed 28 Aug 2025.
5. National Public Radio. The Purdue Pharma deal would deliver billions, but individual payouts will be small. https://www.npr.org/2021/09/28/1040447650/payouts-purdue-pharma-settlement-sackler. Accessed 28 Aug 2025.
6. American Cancer Society. New report: states continue to shortchange tobacco prevention programs, but several show a welcome increase. https://www.fightcancer.org/releases/new-report-states-continue-shortchange-tobacco-prevention-programs-several-show-welcome. Accessed 1 Mar 2025.
7. U.S. Department of Health and Human Services. Office of the Assistant Secretary for Planning and Evaluation. What is lived experience? https://aspe.hhs.gov/sites/default/files/documents/5840f2f3645ae485c268a2784e1132c5/What-Is-Lived-Experience.pdf. Accessed 27 Aug 2025.
8. Falkner R. Engaging with people with lived experience in opioid settlement decision-making. National Academy of State Health. https://nashp.org/engaging-with-people-with-lived-experience-in-opioid-settlement-decision-making/. Accessed 1 Mar 2025.
9. Wisconsin Department of Health Services. Dose of reality: opioids in Wisconsin. https://www.dhs.wisconsin.gov/opioids/index.htm. Accessed 24 Sept 2024.
10. Wisconsin Department of Health Services. Dose of reality: opioid settlement funds. https://www.dhs.wisconsin.gov/opioids/settlement-funds.htm. Accessed 1 Mar 2025.
11. Kaiser Family Foundation Health News. Meet the people deciding how to spend $50 billion in opioid settlement cash. https://kffhealthnews.org/news/article/opioid-settlement-funds-state-council-members-database/. Accessed 29 Aug 2025.
12. Johns Hopkins Bloomberg School of Public Health. The principles for the use of funds from the opioid litigation. https://opioidprinciples.jhsph.edu. Accessed 27 Aug 2025.
13. Johns Hopkins Bloomberg School of Public Health. Nine core strategies. https://opioidprinciples.jhsph.edu/national-dashboard/. Accessed 27 Aug 2025.
14. Putnam-Hornstein E. Why is National child welfare leadership silent on child deaths? https://imprintnews.org/opinion/why-is-national-child-welfare-leadership-silent-on-child-deaths/252134. Accessed 18 Jan 2025.

Conclusion

10

Opioids have taken a devastating toll on America's children and families. What began in the late 1990s as a crisis primarily affecting adults has evolved into a multigenerational tragedy that now claims the lives of individuals across the lifespan, from infants to older adults. The statistics are sobering: more than 600,000 adults and 15,000 children have died from opioid poisonings in the United States since the epidemic began. Behind every statistic is a family that is forever changed by a tragedy.

The lack of attention to children in our national response has been a catastrophic oversight. The impact of the crisis on children has been consistently marginalized in policy discussions, research efforts, and resource allocation.

The core finding from my research over the years is simple but profound: opioid safety must be acknowledged as a family issue rather than an individual one. When an adult brings opioids into the home—whether they are prescribed for pain, medication-assisted treatment, or obtained illicitly—everyone in the household is placed in danger. Our fragmented approach to healthcare in general, and addiction treatment specifically, fails to acknowledge this fundamental reality.

This oversight reflects deeper societal values and institutional structures that often separate adult treatment from child safety. The consequences of this fragmented approach have been devastating: even though thousands of children have died and countless others have been hospitalized, millions more continue to live in homes where opioids are not treated with even basic safety measures.

Our current response has been characterized by well-intentioned but ultimately insufficient measures. Prescription drug monitoring programs address physician prescribing without considering whether the opioids were prescribed according to clinical practice guidelines. Medication-assisted treatment for opioid use disorder undoubtedly saves adult lives but fails to address how these drugs may harm children. Similarly, naloxone expansion focuses on adult overdose reversal without ensuring that families know that the drug can also be used for their children. And finally, Plans of Safe Care for infants exposed in utero to opioids lack meaningful enforcement mechanisms and frequently fail to protect the child.

The medical community shares responsibility for these shortcomings and half-measures. Throughout my research interviewing healthcare providers, I have seen a troubling pattern surrounding knowledge of opioid safety and a misunderstanding of who is responsible for educating families about the risks these drugs pose. Pediatricians assume adult providers are engaging in these conversations with families, while adult providers do not believe that child safety is within their scope of care. Neither provider feels accountable for ensuring that families receive the education they need to truly understand the risks that opioids pose to their children or how to mitigate them.

The data presented throughout this book points to an urgent truth: the home environment is where most pediatric opioid exposures occur and, therefore, where our prevention efforts must focus. This does not diminish the importance of larger systemic changes—indeed, the international examples from Germany, Japan, and the Nordic countries demonstrate that comprehensive, integrated approaches yield the best outcomes for society at large. But it does shift our attention to practical, immediate interventions that could save lives while broader reforms take shape.

Moving forward, I believe we need a fundamental paradigm shift in how we conceptualize the opioid crisis and our response to it. This will necessitate placing families and the interconnectedness of adult and child well-being at the center of our efforts. With billions of dollars in settlement funds now available in states and communities across the United States, we have an opportunity to address the failures and correct historical oversights. However, my analysis of current allocation decisions shows that advisory committees rarely include child advocates or parents who have lost children to opioids. The programs being funded, like Wisconsin's Dose of Reality campaign, fail to adequately address children and family safety. We must ensure that parents and child advocates have a seat at the table.

Thirty years after the opioid crisis began, no one in America should lack a basic understanding of the risks of opioids, how they should be stored, and what to do in case of an emergency. Every household with opioids should have both physical safeguards like lockboxes and knowledge safeguards like emergency response training. These commonsense measures would not only protect children but would likely reduce adult exposures as well.

I began this book by noting that my goal was to shift our current paradigm from one that focuses exclusively on adults to a more systemic, family-centered perspective. The home is where most opioid exposures happen, where prevention is possible, and where practical solutions can have an immediate impact. By embracing this reality, we can build stronger defenses not just against today's opioid crisis but against the future threats that new substances will inevitably bring.

The thousands of families who have lost children to opioids deserve this shift in our collective thinking. By returning to the foundational principles of child safety, family well-being, and shared responsibility, we can finally address this crisis with the comprehensive approach it has always warranted.

Index

A
Accidental addiction, 4, 45
Addiction treatment integration, 95, 96
Adult-centered approaches, 106, 107
Advisory committees, 106, 110
Alcohol, 106
American Academy of Pediatrics (AAP), 73
American Pain Society, 55, 97
America's changing approach, 96, 97
At-home disposal methods, 75

B
Balanced regulatory frameworks, 98

C
Cancer pain, 5
Central nervous system depression, 45
Child Abuse Prevention and Treatment Act (CAPTA) Plan of Safe Care, 46, 60, 81
Child advocates, 106
Child-centered approach, 70
Child Death Review (CDR), 64, 65
Child protection system, 60
Child Protective Services (CPS), 23, 24, 49, 59
Child-resistant packaging, 83
Child safety, 109
Chronic pain, 6, 93, 94
Cognitive-behavioral therapy, 97
Communication training, 72
Community-based support networks, 83
Community dialogue, 105
Community organizations, 75
Community Take-Back Programs, 75
Comprehensive Addiction and Recovery Act, 60
Connecticut law, 46
Conservative prescribing norms, 3
Consumer Product Safety Commission (CPSC), 84
Controlled prescribing practices, 92–94
COVID, 44
Cultural attitudes, 96
Cultural factors, 96

D
Demographic shifts, 41
Department of Children and Families [DCF], 47, 80
Department of Health and Human Services (HHS), 95
Disposal safety, 75
Dose of Reality initiative, 105
Drug, 106

E
Eat, sleep, console approach, 26–28
Education, 70, 71
Electronic health records, 82
Emergency preparedness, 76, 77
ESC model, 27
e-training modules, 95
European Union, 92–93
Evidence-based prescribing guidelines, 98
Evidence-based protections, 107
Evidence-based quality of care, 82
Exposure, 59

F
Family care plans, 60
Family-centered addiction treatment and integrated models, 85, 86
Family-centered models, 98

Family-centered solutions, 106
Family-centered treatment models, 86
Family-focused framework, 69
Family protection
   checklist, 80, 81
   community-based support networks, 83
   evidence-based quality of care and monitoring, 82
   family-centered addiction treatment and integrated models, 85, 86
   healthcare systems integration, 81, 82
   individual households, 79, 80
   regulatory approaches, 83, 84
Family recovery plans, 60
Family support, provider education, 71–73
Fentanyl, 11, 16, 17, 42, 43
Finnegan approach, 21, 26
Finnegan Neonatal Abstinence Scoring Tool (FNAST), 25
Fragmented approach, 109
Funds
   decisions, 103
   distribution and mechanisms, 102, 103

G
Germany, 93

H
Harrison Narcotic Act, 3
Healthcare institutions, 75
Healthcare providers, 71, 104
   knowledge gaps, 60, 61
Healthcare system, 97
   structure of, 94, 95
Heroin, 2, 3
   poisonings, 55
   prescription void, 15, 16
Home-based safety measures, 79
Home-based substance use treatment, 47
Home environment, 110
Homicide, 45, 46

I
Illegally-Manufactured Fentanyl (IMF), 16
Insurance coverage, 98
Integrated care models, 30, 32, 33
Intervention approach, 97

J
Japan's National Healthcare System, 94

Joint Commission on Accreditation of Hospital Organizations (JCAHO), 6

K
KIDOs (Kids in Danger of Opioids) initiative, 83

L
Leung citation, 4

M
Mail-Back Programs, 75
Maternal Overdose Matters (MOMs) Project, 72, 83
Matrix Model for families, 85
Medicaid, 85
Medical community, 110
Medication assisted treatment (MAT), 58
Milligrams of morphine equivalents (MMEs), 13
Morphine, 2
   opioids, initial search, 1
Mothering from the Inside Out (MIO), 85
Multigenerational tragedy, 109
Multi-level prevention strategies, 63

N
Naloxone, 32, 63, 64, 72, 73, 76, 103, 109
National Poison Control Data, 44
National Public Radio (NPR), 107
National Settlement, 101, 103
National Survey on Drug Use and Health (NSDUH), 95
Neonatal opioid withdrawal syndrome (NOWS), 21, 46, 72
   clinical and economic impact of, 22, 23
   eat, sleep, console approach, 26–28
   integrated care models, 30, 32, 33
   long-term challenges for infants with, 23, 24
   prescription and illicit drugs, 21, 22
   research gaps and future directions, 28–30
   standards of care, 25, 26

O
OB-GYN providers, 72
Office of the Child Advocate (OCA), 46, 48
Opioid addiction, 93
Opioid crisis, 107
   America's health disparities, 92

Opioid epidemic
　circumstances and classifications, 45, 46
　Marcello's preventable death, 46–48
　morbidity and mortality findings, 36, 37
　national hospitalization data, mortality record, 35
　pediatric opioid exposures, changing patterns, 38–45
　policy and practice, implications for, 50
　system failures and missed opportunities, 48–50
　victims, 35
Opioid monitoring, racial disparities, 57
Opioid poisonings, national trends, pediatric hospitalization, 37–39
Opioid-related mortality, 92
Opioids, 62
　child-centered approach, 70
　citations, number and type of, 5
　early regulation, 3–6
　education, 70, 71
　family-focused framework, 69
　heroin, 2, 3
　history, 1
　morphine, initial search, 1
　oxycontin, 7–9
　pain as the 5th vital sign, 6, 7
　pediatric deaths, national trends in, 40, 41, 44
　practical home-safety measures, 73, 74
　　emergency preparedness, 76, 77
　　safe disposal, 75, 76
　　storage safety, 74, 75
　risks, 110
　support families, provider education to, 71–73
Opioid safety, 109, 110
　international approaches to, 91, 92
Opioid settlement funds, 101–104, 107
Opioid Settlement Remediation Advisory Committee, 102
Opioid use disorder (OUD), 14, 105
　medication-assisted treatment, 109
Oxycodone, 94
Oxycontin, 1, 4, 7–9, 11, 102
　aftermath of, 11–13
　reformulation of, 14, 15

P
Pain management approaches, 94, 97
Parental education, 71
Pediatric opioid exposures, changing patterns, 38–45

Permanent drop boxes, 75
Plans of safe care (POSC), 60, 81, 109
Poison Control Centers, 62
Poison Prevention Packaging Act (PPPA), 84
Polyethylene oxide, 14
Practical home-safety measures, 73, 74
　emergency preparedness, 76, 77
　safe disposal, 75, 76
　storage safety, 74, 75
Prenatal substance exposure, 106–107
Prescribing practices, 97
Prescription drug monitoring programs, 109
Protection, 80
Provider training, 95, 96
Public health, 11, 16
　messaging, 61, 62
Purdue Pharma, 14
Pure Food and Drug Act, 3

Q
Quality of care, 55, 56, 82

R
Readmission patterns, 32
Residential programs, 85

S
Safety Net
　checklist, 80, 81
　community-based support networks, 83
　evidence-based quality of care and monitoring, 82
　family-centered addiction treatment and integrated models, 85, 86
　healthcare systems integration, 81, 82
　individual households, 79, 80
　regulatory approaches, 83, 84
Safety plans, 60
Settlement agreement, 102
Settlement funds, 107
　opioid, 101, 102
Sober caregiver, 47
Social determinants, 14, 18
Standardized pain assessment protocols, 98
Standard of care, 25, 26
Substance Abuse and Mental Health Services Administration (SAMHSA), 95
Substance use, 49, 97, 103, 104
Substance use disorders (SUDs)., 56, 57, 95, 97, 106, 107
Suicide, 45

Synthetic opioids, 42
Systemic crisis, 53
    emergency preparedness and public health messaging, 61, 62
    failed policy initiatives, 54, 55
    fragmented response, 53, 54
    healthcare provider knowledge gaps and displacement of responsibility, 60, 61
    heightened risks with substance use disorders, 56, 57
    multi-level prevention strategies, 63
    opioid monitoring, racial disparities in, 57
    practices, prioritize adults over children, 59, 60
    quality of care, 55, 56
    regulatory failures, 58, 59
    research and surveillance, 64, 65

T
Tobacco Master Settlement Agreement, 102
Tramadol, 94

U
Universal Insurance Coverage, 94, 95
U.S. opioid epidemic, 11
    changing demographics, 17, 18
    fentanyl, 16, 17
    first wave, availability and deaths, 13, 14
    OxyContin
        aftermath of, 11–13
        reformulation of, 14, 15
    second wave, heroin fills prescription void, 15, 16
    social determinants and vulnerable populations, 14, 18

W
Wisconsin DHS website, 104
Wisconsin initiative, 105
Wisconsin's approach, 106
Wisconsin's community engagement model, 104
Wisconsin's exemplary approach, 105
World Health Care Organization, 30

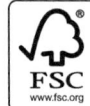

MIX
Papier aus verantwortungsvollen Quellen
Paper from responsible sources
FSC® C105338

If you have any concerns about our products,
you can contact us on
ProductSafety@springernature.com

In case Publisher is established outside the EU,
the EU authorized representative is:
Springer Nature Customer Service Center GmbH
Europaplatz 3, 69115 Heidelberg, Germany

Printed by Libri Plureos GmbH
in Hamburg, Germany